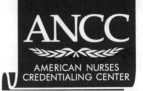

Pediatric nursing review and resource manual.

NURSING REVIEW AND RESOURCE MANUAL

Pediatric Nursing

Published by American Nurses Credentialing Center
Authors: Paula K. Chiplis, PhD, RN, CPNP
Karen Corlett, MSN, RN-BC, CPNP-AC/PC, PNP-BC
Mary Jo Gilmer, PhD, MBA, CNS, CNL
Clara J. Richardson, MSN, RN-BC

CONTINUING EDUCATION SOURCE

NURSING CERTIFICATION REVIEW MANUAL

CLINICAL PRACTICE RESOURCE

2ND EDITION

Rev. ed. of: Pediatric nursing review manual / Joyce Harris. 2002.
Includes bibliographical references and index.
ISBN-13: 978-1-935213-03-1
ISBN-10: 1-935213-03-2
1. Pediatric nursing--Examinations, questions, etc. 2. Pediatric nursing--Outlines, syllabi, etc. I. Chiplis, Paula. II. Harris, Joyce, RN. Pediatric nursing review manual. III. American Nurses Credentialing Center. Institute for Credentialing Innovation.
[DNLM: 1. Pediatric Nursing--methods--United States--Examination Questions. 2. Pediatric Nursing--methods--United States--Handbooks. 3. Pediatric Nursing--methods--United States--Outlines. WY 18.2 P3716 2010]
RJ245.P427 2010
618.92'00231--dc22

2010003303

The American Nurses Credentialing Center (ANCC), a subsidiary of the American Nurses Association (ANA), provides individuals and organizations throughout the nursing profession with the resources they need to achieve practice excellence. ANCC's internationally renowned credentialing programs certify nurses in specialty practice areas; recognize healthcare organizations for promoting safe, positive work environments through the Magnet Recognition Program® and the Pathway to Excellence ® Program; and accredit providers of continuing nursing education. In addition, ANCC's Institute for Credentialing Innovation provides leading-edge information and education services and products to support its core credentialing programs.

ISBN 13: 978-1-935213-03-1
ISBN 10: 1-935213-03-2
© 2010 American Nurses Credentialing Center.
8515 Georgia Ave., Suite 400
Silver Spring, MD 20910

Pediatric Nursing
Review and Resource Manual,
2nd Edition

JANUARY 2010

Please direct your comments and/or queries to: revmanuals@ana.org

The healthcare services delivery system is a volatile marketplace demanding superior knowledge, clinical skills, and competencies from all registered nurses. Nursing autonomy of practice and nurse career marketability and mobility in the new century hinge on affirming the profession's formative philosophy, which places a priority on a lifelong commitment to the principles of education and professional development. The knowledge base of nursing theory and practice is expanding, and while care has been taken to ensure the accuracy and timeliness of the information presented in the **Pediatric Nursing Review and Resource Manual, 2nd Edition**, clinicians are advised to always verify the most current national guidelines and recommendations and to practice in accordance with professional standards of care used with regard to the unique circumstances that apply in each practice situation. In addition, the editors wish to note that provision of information in this text does not imply an endorsement of any particular products, procedures or services.

Therefore, the authors, editors, American Nurses Association (ANA), American Nurses Association's Publishing (ANP), American Nurses Credentialing Center (ANCC), and the Institute for Credentialing Innovation cannot accept responsibility for errors or omissions, or for any consequences or liability, injury, and/or damages to persons or property from application of the information in this manual and make no warranty, express or implied, with respect to the contents of the **Pediatric Nursing Review and Resource Manual, 2nd Edition**.

Published by:
American Nurses Credentialing Center
The Institute for Credentialing Innovation
8515 Georgia Avenue, Suite 400
Silver Spring, MD 20910-3402
www.nursecredentialing.org

Introduction to the Continuing Education (CE) Contact Hour Application Process for *Pediatric Nursing Review and Resource Manual, 2nd Edition*

The Institute for Credentialing Innovation now offers the continuing education contact hours for this manual online at www.NursingWorld.org, the American Nurses Association's Web site. This process involves answering approximately 25–30 questions that test knowledge of the information contained within this manual. The continuing education contact hours can be completed at any time and a certificate can be printed from the Web site immediately upon successful completion of the test.

After studying the manual and given an online multiple-choice test, the exam candidate will be able to:
1. Pass the posttest with at least 75% of the answers correct.
2. Select responses to test questions based on key principles, standards of practice, and theoretical basis of nursing practice.
3. Choose accepted therapeutic interventions in answering questions related to quality nursing practice.
4. Utilize direct and indirect professional role responsibilities and applications regarding nursing practice in answering test questions.

Upon completion of this manual and the online CE test, a nurse can receive a total of 21 continuing education contact hours at a price of $42, only $2 per CE. (ANA members receive a discount on CEs.) The entire process—online test and evaluation form—must be completed by December 31, 2011 in order to receive credit. **To begin the process, please e-mail revmanuals@ana.org.** Your patience with this process is greatly appreciated.

Inquiries or Comments

If you have any questions about the CE contact hours, please e-mail The Institute at revmanuals@ana.org. You may also mail any comments to Editor/Project Manager, at the address listed below.

Duplicate CE Certificates

Once you have successfully passed the CE test on NursingWorld, you may go back and re-print your certificate as often as you wish.

Conflicts of Interest

A conflict of interest occurs when an individual has an opportunity to affect educational content about health-care products or services of a commercial company with which she/he has a financial relationship.

The planners and presenters of this CNE activity have disclosed no relevant financial relationships with any commercial companies pertaining to this activity.

The Institute for Credentialing Innovation
American Nurses Credentialing Center, Attn: Editor/Project Manager
8515 Georgia Avenue, Suite 400
Silver Spring, MD 20910-3492
Fax: (301) 628-5342

The American Nurses Association is accredited as a provider of continuing nursing education by the American Nurses Credentialing Center's Commission on Accreditation.
ANA is approved by the California Board of Registered Nursing, Provider Number 6178.

Contents

Pediatric Nursing
Review and Resource Manual

Taking the Certification Examination

When you sign up to take a national certification exam, you will receive a packet of information from the testing agency. Review it carefully and keep it where you can refer to it frequently. It will contain information on test content and sample questions. This is critical information; review it carefully and it will give you insight into the nature of the test. The agency also will send you materials authorizing your entry into the exam. Keep these in a safe place until needed.

GENERAL SUGGESTIONS FOR PREPARING FOR THE EXAM

Step One: Control Your Anxiety
Everyone experiences anxiety when faced with the certification exam.
- Remember, your program was designed to prepare you to take this exam.
- Your instructors took a similar exam, and have probably talked to students who took exams more recently, so they know how to help you prepare.
- Taking a review course or setting up your own study plan will help you feel more confident about taking the exam.

Step Two: Do Not Listen to Gossip About the Exam

A large volume of information exists about the tests based on reports from people who have taken the exams in the past. Because information from the testing facilities is limited, it is hard not to listen to this gossip.

- Remember that gossip about the exam that you hear from others is not verifiable.
- Because this gossip is based on the imperfect memory of people in a very stressful situation, it may not be very accurate.
- People tend to remember those items testing content with which they are less comfortable; for instance, those with a limited background in women's health may say that the exam was "all women's health." In fact, the exam blueprint ensures that the exam covers multiple content areas without overemphasizing any one.

Step Three: Set Reasonable Expectations for Yourself

- Do not expect to know everything.
- Do not try to know everything in great detail.
- You do not need a perfect score to pass the exam.
- The exam is designed for a beginner level—it is testing readiness for entry-level practice.
- Learn the general rules, not the exceptions.
- The most likely diagnoses will be on the exam, not questions on rare diseases or atypical cases.
- Think about the most likely presentation and most common therapy.

Step Four: Prepare Mentally and Physically

- While you are getting ready to take the exam, take good physical care of yourself.
- Get plenty of sleep, exercise, and eat well while preparing for the exam.
- These things are especially important while you are studying and immediately before you take the exam.

Step Five: Access Current Knowledge

General Content
- You will be given a list of general topics that will be on the exam when you register to take the exam. In addition, examine the table of contents of this book and the test content outline, available at www.nursecredentialing.org/cert/TCOs.html.
- What content do you need to know?
- How well do you know these subjects?

Take a Review Course
- Taking a review course is an excellent method of assessing your knowledge of the content that will be included in the exam.
- If you plan to take a review course, take it well before the exam so you will have plenty of time to master any areas of weakness the course uncovers.
- If you are prepared for the exam, you will not hear anything new in the course. You will be familiar with everything that is taught.
- If some topics in the review course are new to you, concentrate on these in your studies.
- People have a tendency to study what they know; it is rewarding to study something and feel a mastery of it! Unfortunately, this will not help you master unfamiliar content. Be sure to use a review course to identify your areas of strength and weakness, then concentrate on the weaknesses.

Depth of Knowledge

- How much do you need to know about a subject?
- You cannot know everything about a topic.
- Remember that the depth of knowledge required to pass the exam is for entry-level performance.
- Study the information sent to you from the testing agency, what you were taught in school, what is covered in this text, and the general guidelines given in this chapter.
- Look at practice tests designed for the exam. Practice tests for other exams will not be helpful.
- Consult your class notes or clinical diagnosis and management textbook for the major points about a disease. Additional reference books can be found online at www.nursecredentialing.org/cert/refs.html.
- For example, with regard to medications, know the drug categories and the major medications in each. Assume all drugs in a category are generally alike, and then focus on the differences among common drugs. Know the most important indications, contraindications, and side effects. Emphasize safety. The questions usually do not require you to know the exact dosage of a drug.

Step Six: Institute a Systematic Study Plan

Develop Your Study Plan

- Write up a formal plan of study.
  - Include topics for study, timetable, resources, and methods of study that work for you.
  - Decide whether you want to organize a study group or work alone.
  - Schedule regular times to study.
  - Avoid cramming; it is counterproductive. Try to schedule your study periods in 1-hour increments.
- Identify resources to use for studying. To prepare for the examination, on your shelf you should have:
  - A good pathophysiology text.
  - This review book.
  - A physical assessment text.
  - Your class notes.
  - Other important sources, including: information from the testing facility, a clinical diagnosis textbook, favorite journal articles, notes from a review course, and practice tests.
  - Know the important national standards of care for major illnesses.
  - Consult the bibliography on the test blueprint. When studying less familiar material, it is helpful to study using the same references that the testing center uses.
- Study the body systems from head to toe.
- The exam emphasizes health promotion, assessment, differential diagnosis, and plan of care for common problems.
- You will need to know facts and be able to interpret and analyze this information utilizing critical thinking.

Personalize Your Study Plan

How do you learn best?

- If you learn best by listening or talking, attend a review course or discuss topics with a colleague.
- Read everything the test facility sends you as soon as you receive it and several times during your preparation period. It will give you valuable information to help guide your study.
- Have a specific place with good lighting set aside for studying. Find a place with no noise or distractions. Assemble your study materials.

Implement Your Study Plan

You must have basic content knowledge. In addition, you must be able to use this information to think critically and make decisions based on facts.

- Refer to your study plan regularly.
- Stick to your schedule.
- Take breaks when you get tired.
- If you start procrastinating, get help from a friend or reorganize your study plan.
- It is not necessary to follow your plan rigidly. Adjust as you learn where you need to spend more time.
- Memorize the basics of the content areas you will be required to know.

Focus on General Material

- Most of what you need to know is basic material that does not require constant updating.
- You do not need to worry about the latest information being published as you are studying for the exam. Remember, it can take 6 to 12 months for new information to be incorporated into test questions.

Pace Your Studying

- Stop studying for the examination when you are starting to feel overwhelmed and look at what is bothering you. Then make changes.
- Break overwhelming tasks into smaller tasks that you know you can do.
- Stop and take breaks while studying.

Work With Others

- Talk with classmates about your preparation for the exam.
- Keep in touch with classmates, and help each other stick to your study plans.
- If your classmates start having anxiety attacks, do not let their anxiety affect you. Walk away if you need to.
- Do not believe bad stories you hear about other people's experiences with previous exams.
- Remember, you know as much as anyone about what will be on the next exam!

Consider a Study Group

- Study groups can provide practice in analyzing cases, interpreting questions, and critical thinking.
- You can discuss a topic and take turns presenting cases for the group to analyze.
- Study groups can also provide moral support and help you keep studying.

Step Seven: Strategies Immediately Before the Exam

Final Preparation Suggestions
- Use practice exams when studying to get accustomed to the exam format and time restrictions.
  - Many books that are labeled as review books are simply a collection of examination questions.
  - If you have test anxiety, such practice tests may help alleviate the anxiety.
  - Practice tests can help you learn to judge the time you should take during an exam.
  - Practice tests are useful for gaining experience in analyzing questions.
  - Books of questions may not uncover the gaps in your knowledge that a more systematic content review text will reveal.
  - If you feel that you don't know enough about a topic, refer to a text to learn more. After you feel that you have learned the topic, practice questions are a wonderful tool to help improve your test-taking skill.
- Know your test-taking style.
  - Do you rush through the exam without reading the questions thoroughly?
  - Do you get stuck and dwell on a question for a long time?
  - You should spend about 45 to 60 seconds per question and finish with time to review the questions you were not sure about.
  - Be sure to read the question completely, including all four answer choices. Choice "a" may be good, but "d" may be best.

The Night Before the Exam
- Be prepared to get to the exam on time.
  - Know the test site location and how long it takes to get there.
  - Take a "dry run" beforehand to make sure you know how to get to the testing site, if necessary.
  - Get a good night's sleep.
  - Eat sensibly.
  - Avoid alcohol the night before.
  - Assemble the required material—two forms of identification, admission card, pencil, and watch. Both IDs must match the name on the application, and one photo ID is preferred. Bring tissues, antacid chews, hard candy, and anything you might want in your pocket.
  - Know the exam room rules.
    - You will be given scratch paper, which will be collected at the end of the exam.
    - Nothing else is allowed in the exam room.
    - You will be required to put papers, backpacks, etc., in a corner of the room, or in a locker.
    - No water or food will be allowed.
    - You will be allowed to walk to a water fountain and go to the bathroom one at a time.

The Day of the Exam
- Get there early. If you are late, you may not be admitted.
- Think positively. You have studied hard and are well-prepared.
- Remember your anxiety reduction strategies.

SPECIFIC TIPS FOR DEALING WITH ANXIETY
- Test anxiety is a specific type of anxiety. Symptoms include upset stomach, sweaty palms, tachycardia, trouble concentrating, and a feeling of dread. But there are ways to cope with test anxiety.
- There is no substitute for being well-prepared.
- Practice relaxation techniques.
- Avoid alcohol, excess coffee, caffeine, and any new medications that might sedate you, dull your senses, or make you feel agitated.
- Take a few deep breaths and concentrate on the task at hand.

FOCUS ON SPECIFIC TEST-TAKING SKILLS
- To do well on the exam, you need good test-taking skills in addition to knowledge of the content and ability to use critical thinking.

ALL CERTIFICATION EXAMS ARE MULTIPLE CHOICE
- Multiple choice tests have specific rules for test construction.
- A multiple choice question consists of three parts: the information (or stem), the question, and the four possible answers (one correct and three distracters).
- Careful analysis of each part is necessary. Read the entire question before answering.
- Practice your test-taking skills by analyzing the practice questions in this book and on the ANCC Web site.

ANALYZE THE INFORMATION GIVEN
- Do not assume you have more information than is given.
- Do not overanalyze.
- Remember, the writer of the question assumes this is all of the information needed to answer the question.
- If information is not given, it is not relevant and will not affect the answer.
- Do not make the question more complicated than it is.

WHAT KIND OF QUESTION IS ASKED?
- Are you supposed to recall a fact, apply facts to a situation, or understand and differentiate between options?
- Read the question thinking about what the writer is asking.
- Look for key words or phrases that lead you (see Figure 1–1). These help determine what kind of answer the question requires.

READ ALL OF THE ANSWERS
- If you are absolutely certain that answer "a" is correct as you read it, mark it, but read the rest of the question so you do not trick yourself into missing a better answer.
- If you are absolutely sure answer "a" is wrong, cross it off or make a note on your scratch paper and continue reading the question.
- After reading the entire question, go back, analyze the question, and select the best answer.
- Do not jump ahead.
- If the question asks you for an assessment, the best answer will be an assessment. Do not be distracted by an intervention that sounds appropriate.

Figure 1-1. Examples of Key Words and Phrases

avoid	first	likely
best	contributing to	of the following
except	appropriate	most consistent with
not	most	
initial	significant	

- If the question asks you for an intervention, do not answer with an assessment.
- When two answer choices sound very good, the best one is usually the least expensive, least invasive way to achieve the goal. For example, if your answer choices include a physical exam maneuver or imaging, the physical exam maneuver is probably the better choice provided it will give the information needed.
- If the answers include two options that are the opposite of each other, one of the two is probably the correct answer.
- When numeric answers cover a wide range, a number in the middle is more likely to be correct.
- Watch out for distracters that are correct but do not answer the question, combine true and false information, or contain a word or phrase that is similar to the correct answer.
- Err on the side of caution.

ONLY ONE ANSWER CAN BE CORRECT
- When more than one suggested answer is correct, you must identify the one that best answers the question asked.
- If you cannot choose between two answers, you have a 50% chance of getting it right if you guess.

AVOID CHANGING ANSWERS
- Change an answer only if you have a compelling reason, such as you remembered something additional, or you understand the question better after rereading it.
- People change to a wrong answer more often than to a right answer.

TIME YOURSELF TO COMPLETE THE WHOLE EXAM
- Do not spend a large amount of time on one question.
- If you cannot answer a question quickly, mark it and continue the exam.
- If time is left at the end, return to the difficult questions.
- Make educated guesses by eliminating the obviously wrong answers and choosing a likely answer even if you are not certain.
- Trust your instinct.
- Answer every question. There is no penalty for a wrong answer.
- Occasionally a question will remind you of something that helps you with a question earlier in the test. Look back at that question to see if what you are remembering affects how you would answer that question.

ABOUT THE CERTIFICATION EXAMS

The American Nurses Credentialing Center Computerized Exam

The ANCC examination is given only as a computer exam, and each exam is different. The order of the questions is scrambled for every test, so even if two people are taking the same exam, the questions will be in a different order. The exam consists of 175 multiple-choice questions.

- 150 of the 175 questions are part of the test and how you answer will count toward your score, 25 are included to refine questions and will not be scored. You will not know which ones count, so treat all questions the same.
- You will need to know how to use a mouse, scroll by either clicking arrows on the scroll bar or using the up and down arrow keys, and perform other basic computer tasks.
- The exam does not require computer expertise.
- However, if you are not comfortable with using a computer, you should practice using a mouse and computer beforehand so you do not waste time on the mechanics of using the computer.
- Know what to expect during the test.
- Each ANCC test question is independent of the other questions.
  - For each case study, there is only one question. This means that a correct answer on any question does not depend on the correct answer to any other question.
  - Each question has four possible answers. There are no questions asking for combinations of correct answers (such as "a and c") or multiple-multiples.
- You can skip a question and go back to it at the end of the exam.
- You cannot mark key words in the question or right or wrong answers. If you want to do this, use the scratch paper.
- You will get your results immediately, and a grade report will be provided upon leaving the testing site.

OTHER RESOURCES

ANCC Web site: www.nursecredentialing.org

ANA Web site: www.nursesbooks.org. Catalog of ANA nursing scope and standards publications and other titles that may be listed on your test content outline

National Guideline Clearinghouse: www.ngc.gov

2

Developmental and Behavioral Sciences

Paula K. Yim Chiplis, PhD, RN, CPNP, and Mary Jo Gilmer, PhD, MBA, CNS, CNL

Children have unique minds, bodies, and needs. Attention to these differences and consideration of psychosocial and physical growth is essential in assessing, analyzing, and planning care for children. In addition, family context and cultural/spiritual dimensions of care impact a child in a multitude of ways; family dynamics, roles, and values should be a part of each plan of care.

PSYCHOSOCIAL, COGNITIVE, AND ETHICAL-MORAL DEVELOPMENT

Psychosocial theorists whose frameworks are useful in pediatric health care are presented below.

Erikson's Life Stages
A widely accepted theory of personality development was presented in 1963 by this Danish-American developmental psychologist and psychoanalyst. His theory of psychosocial development emphasizes healthy growth through eight stages. Through identification of key conflicts or critical periods in personality development, Erikson described a favorable and unfavorable aspect of each psychosocial stage (Table 2–1).

Table 2-1. Erikson's Life Stages

Age	Psychosocial Stage
Infant (0–12 months)	Trust vs. mistrust
Toddler (1–3 years)	Autonomy vs. shame, doubt
Preschooler	Initiative vs. guilt
School Age	Industry vs. inferiority
Adolescent	Identity vs. role confusion

Piaget's Levels of Cognitive Development

A well-known theory of cognitive development was described by the Swiss developmental psychologist, Jean Piaget. According to Piaget, cognitive development consists of age-related changes that occur in an orderly and sequential manner (Table 2–2).

Through assimilation, children incorporate new knowledge, skills, idea, and insights into their familiar cognitive schemas. Through accommodation, children change and organize existing schemas to solve increasingly difficult tasks.

Maslow's Hierarchy of Needs

Maslow theorized that human needs are hierarchical and the higher levels can only be met when the lower ones are satisfied. The first four needs are basic or "deficiency needs." Self-actualization is a growth need.

- Physiological needs include breathing, food, water, sex, sleep, homeostasis, excretion.
- Safety needs include security of body, employment, resources, morality, family, health, property.
- Love and belongingness needs include friendship, family, sexual intimacy.
- Ego and esteem needs include self-esteem, confidence, achievement, respect for others, respect by others.
- Self-actualization needs include morality, creativity, spontaneity, problem-solving, lack of prejudice, acceptance of facts.

Table 2-2. Piaget's Levels of Cognitive Development

Age	Cognitive Stage	Characteristics
0–2 years	Sensorimotor	Learns through senses and motor activity. Object permanence (something exists even when out of sight) develops and is a basis for stranger anxiety.
2–7 years	Preoperational	Egocentrism shifts to social awareness, magical thinking, and animism. Play is essential as a way of understanding the world and working out experiences.
7–11	Concrete	Understands cause and effect and conservation of matter.
11–15	Formal	Achieves intellectual thought with abstract thinking and ability to consider different outcomes.

Kohlberg's Moral Development

This theory is based on cognitive developmental theory and consists of three major levels. The theory allows for prediction of behavior, but does not consider individual differences.

- Pre-conventional (4–7 yrs). Decisions are based on obedience and avoiding punishment. Morality is external as children conform to rules imposed by authority figures. Present in children and adults.
- Conventional (7–11 yrs). Children are concerned with conformity and being loyal. Rules are to be followed to "be good." Present in teens and adults.
- Post-conventional (≥12 yrs). Internalized standards and social responsibility are formed. Decision can be made in conflicting ethical situations.

BEHAVIOR MODIFICATION

The philosophy and techniques of behavior modification are designed to increase adaptive behavior through positive reinforcement and decrease maladaptive behavior by punishing or ignoring the behavior. For example, a toddler refusing food can learn to eat when reinforced with minutes of playtime for bites of food. Behavior modification is based on the "operant conditioning" principle of learning, also known as Pavlovian and classical conditioning. Basic assumptions include:

- Problems are defined in terms of measurable behavior.
- Treatment is aimed at altering a person's current environment to help the person function in the desired manner.
- Outcome behaviors are specified.
- Methods of treatment and rationale are precisely described.
- Techniques are applied to behaviors of everyday life: toilet training, eating, accepting responsibility for self-care.
- Expected behaviors must be clearly explained and rewards must be attractive enough to reinforce desired behavior.

PHYSICAL DEVELOPMENT: NORMAL GROWTH EXPECTATIONS & DEVELOPMENTAL MILESTONES

Growth is defined as an increase in physical size. Development is an orderly series of events and behaviors that lead to new patterns of behavior. Primary factors influencing growth and development include:

- Genetics
- Nutrition
- Prenatal and environmental factors
- Family and community
- Culture

Preterm (Gestational Age <37 Weeks)

- Minimal subcutaneous fat
- Relaxed posture with limbs extended
- Proportionately large head reflecting cephalocaudal development
- Smooth and shiny skin with visible blood vessels

- Abundant fine lanugo on body
- Soft, pliable ear cartilage (pinnae)
- Palms and soles have minimal creases
- Skull and ribs feel soft
- Head is subject to "premie head," positional molding that can be minimized by frequent repositioning and use of a gel mattress
- Scarf sign—preterm elbow is easily brought across chest

Newborn (Neonate, birth to 28 days)
- **Respiratory system:** Chemical and thermal stimuli initiate respirations. Surface tension of fluid is reduced by surfactant, which facilitates breathing. Respirations are shallow and irregular.
- **Circulatory system:** Inspired oxygen dilates pulmonary vessels, which decreases pulmonary vascular resistance and increases pulmonary blood flow. Ductus arteriosus closes as a result of increased oxygen and decreased prostaglandins. Foramen ovale closes with compression of two portions of atrial septum.
- **Thermoregulation:** Heat regulation is important because of the neonate's large body surface area, thin layer of subcutaneous fat, and lack of shivering.
- **Fluid and electrolytes:** Rapid metabolism can lead to acidosis. Immature kidneys can't concentrate urine well.
- **Gastrointestinal (GI) system:** Deficiency of lipase limits ability to absorb fats. Immature liver decreases storage of glycogen and makes newborn prone to hypoglycemia. Regurgitation and frequent stooling are common.
- **Renal:** Decreased ability to concentrate urine, voids ~200–300 cc/day.
- **Integumentary:** Plugging of sebaceous glands causes milia. Low melanin causes light skin.
- **Musculoskeletal:** Mostly cartilage rather than bone.

Infant (1 to 12 months)
Period of most rapid growth of an individual. Typically, an infant:
- Doubles birth weight by 6 months
- Triples weight by 12 months
- Grows approximately 9–11 inches in first year
- Erupts first tooth at ~6 months
- Needs breast milk or formula for first year of life
- Begins solid foods at 4–6 months, starting with rice cereal
- Posterior fontanelle closes at 6–8 weeks

Milestones of development typically occur in order:
- 1 month: Head lag, grasp reflex strong, hands closed, quiets when hears a voice, fixes on an object at 8–10 inches away, cries and makes comfort noises, watches faces intently
- 2 months: Posterior fontanel fuses, lifts head when prone, visually searches for sounds, cries are differentiated, social smile
- 3 months: Focuses on an object with both eyes (binocular vision), regards own hand, hands loosely open, squeals to show pleasure, coos, babbles, interest in surroundings, aware of strange surroundings
- 4 months: Holds head erect in vertical position, rolls from back to side, grasps objects with both hands, makes consonant sounds (n, k, g, p, b), recognizes familiar faces and objects

- 4–6 months: Sits with support, grasps objects with palm, rolls from stomach to back, plays with toes, grasps and manipulates small objects, prefers complex visual stimuli
- 6 months: Rolls from back to stomach, may chew and bite, begins to imitate sounds, begins to fear strangers, searches for dropped object (concept of object permanence begins), laughs when head is hidden
- 7–8 months: Sits erect momentarily, beginning pincer grasp, reaches for toys out of reach, responds to "no," bears weight on feet with support
- 8–9 months: Crawls on hands and knees, pulls self to standing, hand dominance evident, responds to simple commands, beginning of fears of going to bed and being left alone
- 10 months: Says "dada"
- 12 months: Walks, drinks from cup
- Infant's play is solitary and favorite toys are mobiles, teething toys, plastic blocks, rattles, unbreakable mirror

Toddler (1 to 3 years)

Physical development slows as the toddler's appetite decreases, but needs a diet high in protein for brain development. A toddler typically:
- Drinks whole milk until the age of 2 years, when 2% milk is recommended
- Gains ~3–5 inches and 5 pounds/year
- Quadruples birth weight by 24 months

By age 2 years, doubling a child's height estimates the approximate adult height. The anterior fontanelle fuses between 12 and 18 months. Psychosocial development includes curiosity, gaining sense of autonomy. A toddler typically:
- Generalizes concepts
- Learns to differentiate self from others
- Learns to tolerate separation from primary caregiver
- Engages in parallel play; favorite toys are manipulation toys, blocks, shapes, telephones, kitchens (imitative play)

Preschooler (3 to 6 years)

Growth continues at about 5 pounds and 3 inches/year.
- Appetite decreases
- Needs ~1,800 cal/day
- Has strong food preferences
- Respiratory movement is principally abdominal or diaphragmatic (as opposed to thoracic) in children younger than 6–7 years old

Development is more refined with increased strength/agility.
- Likes to explore
- 3 years: Rides tricycle, copies circle
- 4 years: Throws ball overhand and catches ball, copies a square
- 5 years: Jumps rope, balances on one foot, ties shoes, uses scissors
- Uses associative and cooperative play with favorite toys being creative, educational

School-Age (6 to 12 years)

During the school-age years, growth in height and weight are slower and steadier than earlier years.

- Gains ~2 inches and 4–5 pounds/year
- Loses deciduous teeth beginning at 6 years, with 26 of the 32 permanent teeth erupting by age 12
- Moves gracefully and is steadier than earlier
- Has more mature GI system, so fewer stomach upsets and better maintenance of blood sugar levels
- Prepubescence occurs at ~9 years in girls and ~10 years in boys

Often called the latency period, the school-age child is typically in a period of relative tranquility.

- Engages in cooperative play
- Has a sense of industry
- Maintains relationships with same-sex peers

Adolescence (12 to 18 years)

Teen years are a period of profound biologic, intellectual, psychosocial, and economic change.

- Goes through puberty (growth spurt, sexual maturation with secondary sex characteristics)
- Refines motor skills
- Blood volume and systolic blood pressure increase
- Lung size increases
- Respiratory rate decreases to adult rate
- Has fine tuning of neural system as support cells brace and nourish the neurons

Adolescent development brings advances in cognition with abstract thinking and increasing emotional independence from parents.

- Engages in increasingly competitive play
- Goes through a period of identity formation
- Uses formal operational thought with abstract reasoning
- Is preoccupied with body image
- Generally conforms to group norms
- Has wide mood swings
- Uses principled moral reasoning

FAMILY CONCEPTS AND ISSUES

Families have been defined in many different ways for many different purposes. A family is the mainstay of society and is described as what an individual considers the family to be. This may but does not necessarily include relationships between dependent children and one or more protective adults. Healthcare personnel and services support the family's strength and competence with family-centered philosophy in caring for the child, recognizing that the family is the constant in the child's life. Five major family structures exist, according to the U.S. Census Bureau:

- Traditional nuclear family, which includes a married couple and biological children
- Nuclear family, which includes two parents who may or may not be married, with their children who may be biological, adopted, step, or foster
- Blended family or household, which includes at least one stepparent, stepsibling, or half-sibling
- Extended family or household, which includes at least one parent, one child, and one or more related or unrelated members; parent–child and sibling relationships may be biologic, step, adoptive, or foster.
- Single-parent family, which is increasingly common and usually headed by a single mother, although fathers may be awarded custody

Family theories are used to describe how families respond to events both within and outside the family. Combinations of theories have relevance for nursing practice as each theory has strengths and limitations.

- **Family systems theory:** A change in one part of the family system affects all other parts of the family; families have periods of rapid changes and growth as well as periods of relative stability.
- **Family stress theory:** Families encounter normative, expected, and unexpected stressors and cope with a range of responses and effectiveness. Coping is using learned cognitive and/or behavioral strategies to relieve stress and families cope and respond to stressors with great variability.
- **Family developmental theory:** Families change over time in similar and consistent ways. Duvall (1977) described eight developmental stages of the family throughout the life span.
  - Beginning family that is a newly married or formed couple
  - Child-bearing family with infant
  - Family with preschoolers
  - Family with school-age children
  - Family with teenagers
  - Family launching young adults
  - Middle-aged family—empty nest
  - Family in retirement and old age

  The age of the oldest child indicates the stage. Each stage helps identify transitions and potential stressors. Norms are also developed for blended (step) families, low-income families, single-parent, dual career families, and divorcing families.
- **Structural-functional theory:** The family's major goal is socialization of the child. Family serves to
  - Meet psychological needs of members,
  - Socialize and help children become productive members of society,
  - Perpetuate the species through reproduction,
  - Work as an economic unit, and
  - Provide for physical necessities.

Families play a vital role in society as they produce and consume goods and services; replace dying members of society; and transmit knowledge, customs, values, and beliefs to the young. In working with children, nurses must include family members in the plan of care; the patient is the family.

CULTURAL/SPIRITUAL DIVERSITY

Culture is the totality of socially transmitted values, behavior patterns, institutions, arts, and other products of human work characteristic of a society that organize the society's childrearing system and are transmitted to the next generation by family. Culture provides the context in which families experience health and illness. To provide holistic care, nurses must be culturally sensitive and develop some understanding and appreciation for the ways culture influences childrearing practices and attitudes toward health.

* **Demographic changes:** More than one in five U.S. children are foreign-born or the child of foreign-born parents due to immigration (Mather, 2007). The migration of people requires nurses to be transcultural in their approach to caring for diverse populations. By 5 years old, children can identify persons belonging to their cultural background. The extent to which cultures tolerate divergence from the norm varies.
* **Ethnicity:** A population differentiated from others by customs, characteristics, language, or similar factors. Differences also may include family structure, language, food preferences, moral codes, and expression of emotion. It is difficult for people to attempt to maintain an identity with a subculture while conforming to values of the larger culture.
* Gender may influence the family's perception of the implication of illness/disability. Male children are valued more than female children in some cultures.
* Nurses need to adapt practices to the health needs of families rather than attempt to change longstanding beliefs.
* Nurses need to listen with the goal of understanding rather than agreement.
* Beliefs about health and illness will likely vary from the values of Western healthcare professionals and healthcare institutions.

Religion and spirituality are often used interchangeably, but spirituality is broader than religion. An individual's orientation dictates a code of morality and influences the family's attitude towards education and male/female role identity. Religion may influence choice of life companion(s), profession, diet, acceptability of healthcare options, and rites at birth, circumcision, illness, and death.

* Religion is an integrated system of beliefs that is associated with a code of morality and often influences the family's attitude toward education, gender role identity, professional aspirations, and food choices.
* Spirituality is often defined as an individual's sense of peace, purpose, and connection to others, and beliefs about the meaning of life. While spirituality may be found and expressed through organized religion, many people find meaning in nature or in relationships.

REFERENCES

Bellmore, A. D., Witkow, M. R., Graham, S., & Juvonen, J. (2004). Beyond the individual: The impact of ethnic context and classroom behavioral norms on victims' adjustment. *Developmental Psychology, 40*(6), 1159–1172.

Berndt, T. J. (2002). Friendship quality and social development. *Current Directions in Psychological Science, 11,* 7–10.

Collins, W. A. (2003). More than a myth: The developmental significance of romantic relationships during adolescence. *Journal of Research on Adolescence, 13,* 1–24.

Dishion, T. J., & Kavanagh, K. (2003). *Intervening in adolescent problem behavior: A family-centered approach.* New York: Guilford Press.

Duvall, E. R. (1977). *Family development* (5th ed.). Philadelphia: J.B. Lippincott.

Erikson, E. H. (1963). *Childhood and society* (2nd ed.). New York: W.W. Norton.

Fabes, R. A., Martin, C. L., & Hanish, L. D. (2003). Young children's play qualities in same-, other-, and mixed-sex peer groups. *Child Development, 74,* 921–932.

Fulton, R. A. B., & Moore, C. M. (1995). Spiritual care of the school-age child with a chronic condition. *Journal of Pediatric Nursing, 10*(4), 224–231.

Gauvain, M. (2001). *The social context of cognitive development.* New York: Guilford Press.

Hawley, P. H. (2003). Strategies of control, aggression and morality in preschoolers: An evolutionary perspective. *Journal of Experimental Child Psychology, 85*(3), 213–235.

Hockenberry, M. J., & Wilson, D. (2007). *Wong's nursing care of infants and children* (8th ed.). St. Louis: Mosby Elsevier.

Mather, M. (2007). *U.S. racial/ethnic and regional poverty rates converge but kids are still left behind.* Retrieved from www.prb.org/Articles/2007/USRacialEthnicAndRegionalPoverty.aspx

3

Communication

Karen Corlett, MSN, RN-BC, CPNP-AC/PC, PNP-BC

Communication is a necessary part of health care. Accurate communication between and among nurses, physicians, other members of the healthcare team, patients, families, and caregivers improves the process and delivery of health care.

We communicate with patients and families at every encounter. Some of our encounters are mundane and some involve sharing of quite personal patient or family information. We communicate when taking a patient history, when conveying what we are doing, and when providing instruction. Communication is important to assess health and disease, and to educate about necessary care. Regardless of what we are communicating, the process and structure of communication is much the same. In order to receive and convey content at its best, the elements of ideal communication should be considered.

CULTURALLY SENSITIVE COMMUNICATION

- Assessment of and respect for
  - Usual healthcare providers and systems
    - Complementary and alternative medicine practices and providers
  - Definition of family
    - Make-up of family
    - Family functioning
  - Decision-making processes within the family

- Attitude toward physical contact
- Eye contact
- Native language and/or dialect
- Gender of caregiver in relation to gender of patient or parent
- Religious preferences
- Tenets or beliefs that impact healthcare choices
- Nurses can improve their cultural sensitivity through personal education regarding cultural beliefs, lifestyle differences, and religious practices
  - Do not assume that skin color implies culture

COMPONENTS OF THERAPEUTIC COMMUNICATION

- Establish rapport
  - Honesty, commitment, and caring
- Build trust
  - Commitment of time and availability
- Show respect
  - Address formally unless given permission to use informal levels of address
  - Assessment, acknowledgement, and respect of culture
- Empathy
  - Understanding of and respect for situation
  - Convey concern and caring
- Active listening
  - Verbal content and nonverbal context
  - Clarification of understanding
  - Listener's nonverbal actions are important cues for speaker
- Feedback
  - Verbal and nonverbal encouragement
  - Clarification of content and meaning of verbal and nonverbal communication
- Managing conflict
  - Goal for both parties to come away feeling satisfied
  - Clarify and acknowledge thoughts and feelings of participants
  - Create alternative solutions
  - Negotiate toward acceptable solution with input from all stakeholders
    - Avoid a win–lose situation
    - Goal is win–win
    - Ideal is situation in which each party feels comfortable with compromises made
- Maintain professional boundaries
  - Challenging due to stress/emotions felt during relationship
  - Limit contact with patient and family outside of workplace
  - Avoid sharing personal information with patients and families
- Therapeutic modes of communication with children
  - Talking and listening
  - Role play, acting
  - Storytelling
  - Artwork, drawing, painting, sculpting
  - Music
  - Humor

COMMUNICATION BARRIERS

- Physical barriers
  - Space between participants
  - Qualities of the room
    - Acoustics
    - Audiovisual equipment
    - Temperature
    - Lighting
    - Arrangement of furniture
  - Noise distractions
  - Sensory impairments
    - Hearing, vision, or speech deficits
      - Dialects and accents
    - Drug or disease effects
  - Medical terminology
- Psychosocial barriers
  - Developmental age or stage
    - Consider regression with stress/illness
  - Personal state
    - Emotional state
    - Preconceived ideas
      - About caregiving role
      - Related to disease or diagnosis
    - Previous experiences
      - With healthcare system
      - With persons with similar diagnosis or needs
    - Personal or societal beliefs
      - Values, morals, judgments
    - Body language, facial expressions

MODES OF COMMUNICATION

- Conveying information
  - Talking, lecturing
    - Inflection, tone, and emphasis influence the message
    - One-on-one, small group, large group
  - Written
  - Audio and/or video recordings
  - Interactive programs
- Nonverbal communication
  - Nonverbal message is just as, or more important than, verbal message
  - Body language
    - Open, relaxed posture (avoid crossed arms and knees)
    - At same level as listener
    - Sitting, standing, or kneeling as appropriate
    - Eye contact within constraints of cultural norms

- – Personal space between speakers and listeners
    - Defined differently among cultures
    - Be aware of physical barriers that may be between speaker and recipients such as crib railings or the hospital bed
- – Appearance
    - Clothing, hairstyle, body art, jewelry, and so on
- – Hand gestures
- – Touch/physical contact
- Receiving information
    - Listening
        - Active process
        - Give feedback regarding degree of understanding
            - Restate
            - Summarize
            - Ask for clarification
- Formal communication
    - Preplanned
    - Organized
    - Objectives predetermined
- Informal communication
    - Just as powerful as formal communication
    - Spontaneous
        - Taking advantage of teachable moments
    - Often occurs during other events/tasks
    - Can be a less intimidating process
        - Fewer barriers
        - Often yields more feelings
- Group dynamics
    - Forming
        - Politeness prevails
        - Getting to know—not much revealed as of yet
        - Group members get along well or pretend to
    - Storming
        - Maneuvering for position within the group
        - Informal role assignments (leader, negotiator, defender, etc.)
        - Attempts at doing the work of the group
    - Norming
        - Trust develops
        - Issues revealed
        - The group starts to work well together
    - Performing
        - Active work predominates
        - Cooperation and efficiency
        - The group works smoothly
    - Adjourning/mourning
        - A formal dissolution of the group
        - Important for participants to sense that the purpose or work of group is completed

– Groups work through these stages at different speeds
  • May spend more time in one stage than another
  • May cycle through all these stages in one efficient meeting
  • Groups that can not get through "norming" rarely perform well

PATIENT CONFIDENTIALITY

• Health Insurance Portability and Accountability Act (HIPAA)
  – National mandate to protect the privacy of patient information
    • Structures in place to protect the privacy of the medical record
    • All written and verbal communication about patient status is protected
    • Computers and portable access devices must have protection in place
  – Appropriate sharing of information
    • Between healthcare providers and family members with patient's permission
    • Among healthcare providers to facilitate safe care
    • Among healthcare entities, billing departments, and insurers
      - Only necessary information should be shared
  – Mandatory reporting
    • Reportable diseases to health departments or government agencies
    • Police reports, such as for gunshot injuries
    • Suspected or documented nonaccidental injury, neglect, abuse

WRITTEN COMMUNICATION IN NURSING PRACTICE

• A part of the medical record
  – Legal document
  – Documentation of nursing care delivered
  – Documentation of patient status
• Timed and dated
  – Entered into record in a timely fashion
• Legible
  – Content and signature
• Accurate
• Use of only approved abbreviations
• Errors corrected appropriately

PROFESSIONAL COMMUNICATION

• With other care team providers
  – Healthcare jargon is appropriate
    • Precise meanings conveyed
• Much of communication is verbal
  – Document important elements of verbal exchanges in the medical record

- Transfer of care
  - When transferring care of patient temporarily or permanently
  - Concise yet complete
  - SBAR
    - Situation
    - Background
    - Assessment
    - Recommendations
      - Include issues, tests, and results that are in process or pending
  - Can be verbal or written process
    - Must have opportunity to clarify information and ask questions as part of transfer of care process
    - SBAR be used for any situation in which information is communicated between members of the healthcare team
- Dealing with difficult people
  - Address behavior privately
    - Away from patient's family members and other patients or families
    - Away from patient care areas if conflict between providers
    - May be helpful to have neutral third party present
  - Describe issue/conflict/behavior
    - Remain calm, use "I" statements
    - Describe effects of words or actions
  - If issues unresolved, escalate concerns via appropriate chain of command
    - Nursing chain of command
    - Family services chain of command
    - Medical staff office chain of command
    - State nurses association

ADVOCACY

- Professional advocacy
  - For the profession of nursing
    - Expand your personal knowledge base
    - Know what it is to be a nurse and how to explain the profession to families and other providers
      - Address myths or incorrect beliefs
    - Differentiate between physician orders and nursing care plans
      - Highlight the practice of nursing
    - Join a professional organization
      - Participate in committees
      - Seek office
    - Contact government representatives in support of the nursing profession
      - Become aware of proposed regulations affecting nurses

– For patients and families
  - Advocate for family-centered care in your facility
  - Provide developmentally appropriate care for the child
  - Support community endeavors beneficial to children's health
  - Lobby for change to support children's health care
    - At the community, state, and national levels
    - Get involved with child advocacy organizations
    - Become aware of and involved with legislative changes

REFERENCES

The Center for Nursing Advocacy. (2003–2008). *Homepage.* Retrieved from www.nursingadvocacy.org

Institute for Healthcare Improvement. (n.d.). *SBAR technique for communication: A situational briefing model.* Retrieved from http://www.ihi.org/IHI/Topics/PatientSafety/SafetyGeneral/Tools/SBARTechniqueforCommunicationASituationalBriefingModel.htm

Potts, N. L., & Mandleco, B. L. (Eds.). (2007). *Pediatric nursing: Caring for children and their families* (2nd ed.). Clifton Park, NY: Tomson.

U.S. Department of Health and Human Services. (2003). *Summary of the HIPAA privacy rule.* Retrieved from http://hhs.gov/ocr/hipaa

4

The Nursing Process

Clara J. Richardson, MSN, RN-BC

The nursing process is a standardized method of identifying client needs/problems and then problem-solving to meet those needs. The six steps of the nursing process are assessment, diagnosis, outcome identification, planning, implementation, and evaluation.

NURSING ASSESSMENT

Assessment of the Child and Family

The pediatric health history may be altered based on setting, age of the child, and focus of care. In the ambulatory setting, the history is extensive and expanded with each visit as the practitioner strives to provide comprehensive well-child care. At the hospital, the focus is on the areas of history most relevant to the present condition. Prenatal and birth history tends to become briefer with older children. Ideally, in an integrated healthcare system, the individual's lifetime health history would be available to all providers in all settings.

Identifying Data
- Child's nickname
- Informant's relationship to the child

Reason for Seeking Care
- Progression of symptoms
- Exposure to communicable disease

Past Medical History
- Immunization record
- Communicable diseases
- Past illnesses, surgeries, hospitalizations, emergency room visits
- Allergies to medications, foods, animals, insects, dust, etc.
- Current medications, vitamins, nutritional supplements

Birth History

PRENATAL HISTORY
- Maternal health
  - Age and extent of prenatal care
  - Past pregnancies
  - Illnesses, exposure to diseases or environmental toxins
  - Attitudes toward the pregnancy
- Maternal medications
  - Prescribed medications
  - Vitamins and over-the-counter medications
  - Illicit drugs, alcohol, smoking
- Length of gestation, problems encountered
- Parents' blood types

NATAL HISTORY
- Labor and delivery
  - Length of labor
  - Spontaneous or induced
  - Vaginal or cesarean
  - Forceps
  - Medications, epidural anesthesia
- Infant's condition at birth
  - Apgar scores
  - Gestational age assessment
  - Birth weight, length, head circumference

NEONATAL HISTORY
- Problems
  - Respiratory problems, jaundice, seizures
  - Thermoregulation or glucose problems
  - Neonatal intensive care unit
  - Any other problems
- Length of hospital stay
- First weeks at home
  - Feeding
  - Sleeping
  - Elimination
- Family bonding
  - Parent–child
  - Siblings
  - Extended family, friends

Dietary History

INFANT FEEDING
- Duration of breastfeeding
- Formula brand, preparation, storage
- Introduction of solids, finger foods
- Vitamin, iron, or fluoride supplements

OLDER CHILD
- Age of weaning from breast or bottle
- Self-feeding skills
- 24-hour recall, usual diet
- Vitamins, nutritional supplements
- Food preferences, foods avoided
- Food allergies

Developmental History

- Developmental milestones

TOILET TRAINING
- Age
- Methods
- Problems

DENTITION
- Number of teeth
- Dental hygiene
- Visits to dentist

SLEEP PATTERNS
- Amount and timing
- Place, bedtime rituals
- Nightmares, terrors, waking

HABITS
- Thumb sucking, nail biting, hair twisting
- Temper tantrums
- Alcohol, drug use, huffing
- Smoking, smokeless tobacco

Social History

RESIDENCE
- Home type, condition, size, safety precautions
- City or well water
- Urban or rural
- Neighborhood, play area safety
- Residents and relationships
- Pets

FINANCIAL SITUATION
- Parents' occupations
- Source of healthcare payment
  - Private insurance
  - Medicaid
- Social agency assistance

FAMILY RELATIONSHIPS
- Family roles and organization
- Languages spoken and read
- Childrearing practices, discipline
- Extended family
- Support systems

COMMUNITY INVOLVEMENT
- Childcare, school
- Social clubs, sports, activities
- Religious involvement

Family Health History
- Ages and health problems
- Genetic or familial health problems

Health Practices
- Usual providers
- Regularity of well-child visits
- Lay providers, folk healers
- Religious practices related to health
- Illness prevention and treatment
  - Special foods, beverages, herbs, spices, supplements
  - Ointments, creams, steam, heat, cold, massage
  - Other forms of complementary and alternative medicine
  - Over-the-counter medications

Physical Assessment

Age Variations and Tips
INFANTS/TODDLERS
- Keep on parent's lap as much as possible
- While quiet do auscultation, pulse, respirations
- Save intrusive activities (temperature, throat, ears) until the end
- Keep security objects near
- Use distraction

PRESCHOOLERS
- Short, simple verbal explanations
- Demonstrate on dolls, stuffed animals
- Let child handle equipment
- Save genitalia until the end

SCHOOL-AGE CHILDREN
- Explain purpose of assessment and body functioning
- Use pictures, body diagrams
- Save genitalia until the end

ADOLESCENTS
- Provide privacy and assure confidentiality
- Keep conversation nonjudgemental, nonconfrontational
- Save genitalia until the end

Growth Measurements

GENDER-SPECIFIC GROWTH CHARTS MAY BE DOWNLOADED FROM THE NATIONAL CENTER FOR HEALTH STATISTICS
- Infants, birth to 36 months
  - Length for age and weight for age
  - Head circumference for age
  - Weight for length
- Children and adolescents, 2–20 years
  - Stature for age and weight for age
  - Body mass index (BMI) for age
- Preschoolers, 2–5 years
  - Weight for stature

HEIGHT
- Length is measured in lying position
- Stature is measured in standing position
- Within normal limits if between 5th and 95th percentiles
- Children should follow a steady curve on standardized growth chart
- Use gestation-adjusted age for premature infants up to 24 months of age when using standardized growth chart

WEIGHT
- Children younger than 3 years weighed nude
- Underwear or light gown for older children
- Within normal limits if between 5th and 95th percentiles
- Children should follow a steady curve on standardized growth chart
- Use gestation-adjusted age for premature infants up to 24 months of age when using standardized growth chart

HEAD CIRCUMFERENCE MEASURED IN CHILDREN UP TO 36 MONTHS

Vital Signs

TEMPERATURE
- Axillary for infants younger than 1 month
- Rectal for infants older than 3 months
- Temporal artery not accurate for infants younger than 3 months with acute illness or fever
- Tympanic more accurate for children older than 6 months
- Oral for cooperative children

PULSE
- Apical for children younger than 2 years
- Count for full minute
- Usual rates
  - Newborn   100–180
  - <2 years   80–130
  - 2–6 years   70–120
  - 6–10 years   70–110
  - 10–16 years   60–100

RESPIRATIONS
- Count for full minute
- Usual rates
  - Newborn   30–60
  - 1 year   20–40
  - 2–5 years   20–30
  - 10 years   16–20
  - 17 years   12–20

BLOOD PRESSURE
- Cuff bladder width 40% of upper-arm circumference
- Cuff bladder length 80%–100% of upper-arm circumference
- Percentile charts available from Centers for Disease Control (www.cdc.gov)
- Estimate of usual value
  - Systolic:
    · Ages 1–7 years = age in years + 90
    · Ages 8–18 years = (2 x age in years) + 83
  - Diastolic:
    · Ages 1–5 years = 56
    · Ages 6–18 years = age in years + 52

Pediatric Variations of Adult Physical Assessment Findings
LYMPH NODES: SMALL, NONTENDER, MOVABLE NODES ARE USUALLY NORMAL IN CHILDREN

HEAD
- Flatness or bald spot on one side or back of head often denotes lying in one position
- Infant should hold head erect and midline by age 4 months
- Anterior fontanel closes at 12–18 months of age

NECK
- Neck short until age 3–4 years
- Any mass can easily obstruct airway

EYES
- Permanent eye color by age 6–12 months
- Presence of red reflex rules out many serious defects

- Infant should be able to fixate on one visual field by age 3–4 months
- Visual acuity testing should begin by age 3 years
    - Snellen letter charts
    - Tumbling E chart
    - HOTV chart
    - Allen picture test

EARS
- For otoscopic exam
    - Pull pinna down and back for children younger than 3 years
    - Pull pinna up and back for children older than 3 years
- Variety of auditory tests for newborns and older children

CHEST
- Children younger than 6 years use abdominal, rather than diaphragmatic, breathing
- Breast changes of puberty start in girls at 10–14 years
- Gynecomastia in boys may be due to hormonal conditions or obesity
- See Chapter 9 for additional respiratory assessment
- See Chapter 10 for additional cardiac assessment

ABDOMEN
- To check for inguinal hernia in child too young to cough, have them blow hard through a straw or laugh

EXTREMITIES
- Absence of femoral pulse may indicate coarctation of the aorta
- Bow-leg appearance is normal in children younger than 3 years
- Knock-knee appearance is normal until 7 years of age

Pain Assessment Tools Based on Age of Child

Premature Infant Pain Profile Scale (PIPPS): Neonates with gestational ages of 28 to greater than 36 weeks gestation
- Gestational age
- Behavioral state
- Heart rate
- Oxygen saturation
- Brow bulge
- Eye squeeze
- Nasolabial furrow

CRIES Scale: 0–6 months
- Crying
- Requires O_2 for SaO_2 <95%
- Increased vital signs (blood pressure and heart rate)
- Expression
- Sleepless

Neonatal Infant Pain Scale (NIPS): <1 year
- Facial expression
- Cry
- Breathing patterns
- Arms
- Legs
- State of arousal

FLACC Scale: 2 months–7 years
- Face
- Legs
- Activity
- Cry
- Consolability

Children's Hospital Eastern Ontario Pain Scale (CHEOPS): 1–7 years
- Cry
- Facial
- Child verbal
- Torso
- Touch
- Legs

Oucher Scale: 3–12 years
- Six photograph faces ranging from not hurt to biggest hurt you could ever have
- White, Black, Hispanic forms

FACES Pain Rating Scale: >3 years
- Six cartoon faces ranging from no hurt to hurts worst
- English and Spanish forms

Non-Communicating Children's Pain Checklist:
3–18 years with cognitive impairment
- Vocal
- Social
- Facial
- Activity
- Body and limbs
- Physiological
- Eating/sleeping

Numeric Pain Scale: >9 years
- None
- Mild: 0–3
- Moderate: 4–6
- Severe: 7–10

COMFORT Scale: Infants, children, adults
- Alertness
- Calmness
- Respiratory distress
- Crying
- Physical movement
- Muscle tone
- Facial tension
- Blood pressure
- Heart rate

Family Assessment Tools

Calgary Family Assessment Model: An in-depth evaluation
- Structural category: Family members, caregivers, supports outside of immediate family
- Developmental category: Life stage events (divorce, childbirth, etc.)
- Functional category: Interaction of family members

Family Adaptability and Cohesion Evaluation Scales IV (FACES IV): In-depth evaluation of balanced (healthy) and unbalanced (problematic) family functioning
- Balanced
- Rigidly cohesive
- Midrange
- Flexibly unbalanced
- Chaotically disengaged
- Unbalanced

Family Apgar: Very brief 5-item scale to measure family members' satisfaction
- Family problem-solving
- Shared responsibility and decision-making
- Physical and emotional maturation, self-fulfillment
- Commitment to share time, space, and material resources

Friedman Family Assessment Model: Variable depth through short and long forms
- Identifying data
- Developmental stage and history
- Environmental data
- Family structure
- Family functions
- Family stress, coping, adaptation

Home Observation for Measurement of the Environment (HOME):
Short and long forms depending on depth
- Measure quality and quantity of stimulation and support available to child in the home
- Infant/Toddler (IT) HOME
- Early Childhood (EC) HOME
- Middle Childhood (MC) HOME
- Early Adolescent (EA) HOME
- Child Care (CC) HOME
- Disability (DA) HOME

NURSING DIAGNOSIS

Nursing diagnosis is a standardized language to communicate client needs/problems, which may be actual or potential problems based on the client's risk factors. The North American Nursing Diagnosis Association (NANDA) produced the first taxonomy in 1986. Renamed NANDA International (http://www.nanda.org/html), the organization remains committed to the continued development of nursing diagnostic terminology.

The Nursing Interventions Classification (NIC) provides a standardized list of more than 500 research-based physiological and psychosocial interventions. The Nursing Outcome Classification (NOC) contains more than 300 outcomes that can be used to evaluate the effects of nursing interventions. These classifications are available from the University of Iowa's Center for Nursing Classification and Clinical Effectiveness at http://www.nursing.uiowa.edu/excellence/nursing_knowledge/clinical_effectiveness/index.htm.

OUTCOME IDENTIFICATION

After identifying the appropriate nursing diagnoses, the nurse specifies the expected changes in physical condition or behavior that the client will exhibit after interventions are implemented. Client outcomes should consist of specific behaviors that can be seen, measured, or evaluated. They should also include a time frame for attainment. Nurses usually develop their own outcomes, but NOC could certainly be used and may provide a usable format for computerized charting.

PLANNING

Once the nurse defines client outcomes, she or he describes specific nursing interventions that will assist the client in attaining those outcomes. Evidence-based interventions come from data the nurse gathers from client's statements, from the nurse's own observations, and from current research information. The nurse uses critical thinking to plan care based on the evidence and her or his own clinical expertise. Searching for evidence requires that the nurse be able to access information using appropriate computer search engines. Again, nurses usually develop their own interventions, but using NIC language may have some advantages if standardization is desired.

IMPLEMENTATION

Implementation is the nurse fulfilling the role of care provider, putting plans into action. It must be noted that all nursing care in pediatrics is family-centered care. The entire family, not just the child, is the client. The nurse implements interventions for all family members to enable them to show their present competencies and develop new competencies with the ultimate goal of empowering families to control their own lives.

EVALUATION

In the evaluation step of the process, the nurse decides if the client outcomes were met, if the nursing interventions were effective, and if the plan needs modification. If alterations are required and the client interaction continues, the last step of the nursing process may not actually be the end.

REFERENCES

Asher, C., & Northington, L. K. (2008). Position statement for measurement of temperature/fever in children. *Journal of Pediatric Nursing, 23,* 234–235.

Breau, L., McGrath, P., Finley, A., & Camfield, C. (2004). *Non-communicating children's pain checklist—revised (NCCPC-R).* Retrieved from http://www.aboutkidshealth.ca/Shared/PDFs/AKH_Breau_everyday.pdf

Caldwell, B., & Bradley, R. (1984). *Home observation for measurement of the environment (HOME) inventory.* Retrieved from http://ualr.edu/case/index.php/home/home-inventory/

Callahan, H. E. (2003). Families dealing with advanced heart failure: A challenge and an opportunity. *Critical Care Nursing, 26,* 230–243.

Faulds, S., & Moore, J. (2007). *Pediatric pain assessment tools.* Retrieved from http://www.anes.ucla.edu/pain/assessment_tools.html

Hockenberry, M. J., & Wilson, D. (2007). *Wong's nursing care of infants and children.* St. Louis, MO: Mosby Elsevier.

Knafl, K. A., Knafl, G. J., Gallo, A. M., & Angst, D. (2007). Parents' perceptions of functioning in families having a child with a genetic condition. *Journal of Genetic Counseling, 16,* 481–492.

Manworren, R. C. B., & Hynan, L. S. (2003). Clinical validation of FLACC: Preverbal patient pain scale. *Pediatric Nursing, 29,* 140–146.

Martin-Arafeh, J. M., & Watson, C. L., & Baird, S. M. (1999). Promoting family-centered care in high risk pregnancy. *The Journal of Perinatal and Neonatal Nursing, 13*(1), 27–42.

Moore, K. A., Halle, T. G., Vandivere, S., & Mariner, C. L. (2002). Scaling back survey scales: How short is too short. *Sociological Methods & Research, 30,* 530–567.

National Center for Health Statistics. (2008). *Clinical growth charts.* Retrieved from http://www.cdc.gov/nchs/about/major/nhanes/growthcharts/clinical_charts.htm

National Institutes of Health. (2007). *Pain intensity instruments.* Retrieved from http://painconsortium.nih.gov/pain_scales/

Olson, D. H., & Gorall, D. M. (2006). *FACES IV & the circumplex model.* Retrieved from http://www.facesiv.com/pdf/3.innovations.pdf

Oucher Organization. (1983). *Oucher!*™ Retrieved from http://www.oucher.org/the_scales.html

Pasero, C. (2002). Pain assessment in infants and young children: Premature infant pain profile. *American Journal of Nursing, 102,* 105–106.

Weitzman, C. C., Roy, L., Walls, T., & Tomlin, R. (2004). More evidence for reach out and read: A home-based study. *Pediatrics, 113,* 1248–1253.

Willis, M. H. W., Merkel, S. I., Voepel-Lewis, T., & Malviya, S. (2003). FLACC behavioral pain assessment scale: A comparison with the child's self-report. *Pediatric Nursing, 29,* 195–198.

5

Basic and Applied Science

Paula K. Yim Chiplis, PhD, RN, CPNP, and
Mary Jo Gilmer, PhD, MBA, CNS, CNL

TRAUMA AND DISEASE PROCESSES

An understanding of age-specific anatomy and physiology, common genetic disorders, transmission of infectious diseases, and the use of traction to treat fractures is essential to the pediatric nurse.

Age-Specific Anatomy and Physiology

Defined and predictable patterns in growth and development are universal to all children, but they follow the patterns in a manner and time that is unique to each child (Hockenberry & Wilson, 2009).

Directional Trends
- Cephalocaudal (head/down)
- Proximal to distal (inside/outside)
- Differentiation (simple/complex)

Biologic Growth
- Skeletal maturation occurs over ~20 years, beginning with centers of ossification in an embryo and concluding when the last epiphysis is fused to the shaft of a bone. Bone fractures may be difficult to discover and may impact subsequent growth and development.

- Neurologic primitive reflexes are replaced by intentional movements as the brain develops. Growth of the brain is reflected in increasing head circumference, possible until fontanelles close.
- Lymphoid tissues are relatively small in infants, but are well-developed and grow quickly.
- Kidneys and liver are immature at birth and in early childhood, leading to decreased metabolism of medications and fairly diluted urine.

Physiological Changes
- Metabolism describes all chemical and energy transformations in the body. Basal metabolic rate (BMR) is slightly higher in boys than in girls and further increases over girls in pubescence.
- Thermoregulation is an important adaptation to extra-uterine life and even young children are susceptible to temperature fluctuations. Infections can result in either a rapid temperature elevation or a decrease in temperature in young children. Young children also can become overheated during active play.

Common Genetic Disorders
Prenatal diagnosis is available for many disorders, leading to ethical dilemmas such as whether to use the option of abortion.
- Cystic fibrosis is an autosomal recessive condition with abnormal exocrine gland function and excessive salt in sweat. Most common lethal disease in Whites; median life span 25 years.
    - Chronic pulmonary involvement: Excessive mucous, reduced cilia function, recurrent infections
    - Pancreatic compromise: Lack of trypsin, malabsorption; also rectal prolapse, meconium ileus, liver cirrhosis, gallbladder tones, salivary gland obstruction
    - Prenatal diagnosis available at chromosome 7q31.2 and sweat chloride test used for postnatal diagnosis
- Sickle cell disease (SCD) is an autosomal recessive, chronic hemolytic anemia from production of abnormal hemoglobin (HbS) with reduced oxygen-carrying capacity. The disease causes infarction of lungs, kidneys, spleen, bones, painful leg ulcers, dactylitis, priapism, renal failure, increased risk for pneumococcal infections and salmonella osteomyelitis. Incidence is 1:400–600 in Blacks. Prenatal diagnosis available at chromosome 11p15.5. Postnatal screening test is Sickledex; electrophoresis provides definitive diagnosis.
- Trisomy 21 (Down syndrome) is compatible with live birth, but physical and mental abnormalities vary greatly. IQ 25–75; 50% die by 60 years; males are sterile. Characterized by mental retardation, craniofacial abnormalities, low-set ears, ventricular and atrial septal defects, patent ductus arteriosus, hypotonia, respiratory infections, acute leukemia, malformed kidneys, hydronephrosis, cryptorchidism, seizures, apneic events. Frequency 1:1,500 for mothers 20 years old and 1:30 for mothers 45 years old. Prenatal and postnatal diagnoses available at chromosome 21.
- Achondroplasia is an autosomal dominant common form of dwarfism; adult stature 48–52 inches. Characterized by shortened limbs, normal-length torso, lordosis, sleep apnea, possible hydrocephalus, prominent forehead, flattened nasal bridge, short stubby fingers, normal IQ and life span; women may have backaches, premature menarche and menopause, enlarged breasts. Prenatal diagnosis available on chromosome 4p16.3.

- Huntington disease is an autosomal dominant, progressive neurological deterioration caused by neuron atrophy with death approximately 15 years from onset. Onset at 15–50 years. Characterized by psychiatric symptoms, choreoathetoid movements, progressive dementia, intellectual decline, seizures, rigidity, and dystonia. Prenatal diagnosis available on chromosome 4p16.3.
- Familial hypercholesterolemia is an autosomal dominant, common single-gene disorder with early onset atherosclerotic disease of coronary, cerebral, and peripheral arteries and xanthomas (cholesterol deposits in skin and tendons); 1:200–500. Diagnosis available on chromosome 19p13.2.
- Osteogenesis imperfecta is an autosomal dominant osteoporosis with recurrent fractures of long bones. Life span normal in spite of repeated fractures. Characterized by blue sclera, conductive deafness, discolored teeth, and multiple fractures. Diagnosis available on chromosome 17q21.31.
- Polycystic kidney disease is an autosomal dominant condition with development of cysts in kidneys, liver, pancreas, and spleen; renal failure; and hypertension. Cysts remain asymptomatic until 3rd or 4th decade; incidence 1:1,000; accounts for 10% of adult cases of renal failure. Diagnosis available on chromosome 4121.

Common Childhood Diseases

Newborn

CONJUNCTIVITIS OF THE NEWBORN (OPHTHALMIA NEONATORUM) < 30 DAYS
- Characteristics: Red conjunctiva, swollen with yellow or white discharge
- Complications: Periorbital cellulitis, brain abscess, and decreased vision
- Treatment: Usually optic antibiotics since the condition is caused by *Chlamydia* and/or *Neisseria gonorrhea*
- Nursing management: Instilling antibiotics, teaching parents careful handwashing, and limiting exposure to other children until on antibiotics for 24 hours

ATOPIC DERMATITIS (ECZEMA)
- Characteristics: Chronic red, pruritic crust or vesicles on face, scalp, and/or extensor aspects of arms and legs
- Complications: Secondary skin infections
- Treatment: Avoid allergy-causing foods and environmental factors; lubricate with moisturizing ointments and creams (Eucerin, Elidel, Aquaphor, Cetaphil, Protopic, Vaseline) 3–4x/day; apply topical steroids (ointment preferred) such as hydrocortisone 1%–2.5%
- Nursing management: Reduce frequency of bathing to a few times/week in tepid, not hot, water; lubricate skin after bathing or swimming; apply hydrocortisone 0.5%–1%; use Benadryl or Atarax for pruritus

Infancy

COW'S MILK ALLERGY (CMA)
- Characteristics: Crying, pallor, irritability, diarrhea, vomiting, colic, wheezing, bloody stools, rhinitis, asthma, sneezing, coughing, and/or eczema within first 4 months of life
- Complications: Slow growth, possible anaphylaxis

- Treatment: Eliminate cow's milk–based formula to a casein hydrolysate milk formula such as Pregestimil, Nutramigen, or Alimentum, in which mild proteins are broken into amino acids
- Nursing management: Reassure and educate parents; maintain infants on a milk-free diet for 1–2 years, after which small quantities of milk are reintroduced; many children outgrow sensitivity by 3–4 years old

DIAPER DERMATITIS
- Incidence is 50% of young children, peak age 9–12 months, and caused by wetness, pH, and fecal irritants; risk factors for Candida albicans infection are altered immune status and antibiotic therapy
- Characteristics: Bright red rash with raised borders, often with satellite lesions in skin folds
- Complications: Scarring, systemic infections
- Treatment: Topical glucocorticoids or antifungals if nursing management not successful
- Nursing management: Superabsorbent disposable diapers, change diapers frequently, expose to air (minor diaper dermatitis) or use thick zinc oxide or petroleum to protect skin (moderate–severe)

Early Childhood

CHICKENPOX (VARICELLA-ZOSTER VIRUS, VZV)
- Transmission: Spread by respiratory secretions and direct contact with skin lesions, although scabs are not infectious; incubation 2–3 weeks
- Characteristics: Rash on trunk with less on limbs
- Complications: Secondary bacterial infections (e.g., abscesses, cellulitis, necrotizing fasciitis, pneumonia, sepsis), encephalitis, hemorrhagic varicella, chronic or transient thrombocytopenia
- Treatment: Antiviral acyclovir and VZIG in high-risk children, diphenhydramine to relieve itching
- Vaccine: Available; see the Center for Disease Control and Prevention's Web site, www.cdc.gov/vaccines
- Nursing management: Isolation until vesicles are dry to prevent spread, daily tepid baths and skin care, calamine lotion, keep fingernails short and clean, keep child cool to decrease itching

DIPHTHERIA (CORYNEBACTERIUM DIPHTHERIAE)
- Transmission: Direct contact with discharge from nose, skin, and lesions
- Characteristics: Fever; malaise; highly pruritic rash that starts as macule and progresses to vesicle that breaks and crusts; lymphadenopathy; pseudomembrane in nasal, pharyngeal or laryngeal areas
- Complications: Myocarditis, neuritis
- Treatment: Penicillin or erythromycin, complete bedrest to prevent myocarditis, tracheostomy for airway obstruction
- Vaccine: Available; see the Center for Disease Control and Prevention's Web site, www.cdc.gov/vaccines
- Nursing management: Maintain isolation, have epinephrine available, observe respirations for obstruction, suction as necessary, administer humidified oxygen

FIFTH DISEASE OR ERYTHEMA INFECTIOSUM (HUMAN PARVOVIRUS B19)

- Transmission: Unknown route, possibly respiratory secretions of infected persons
- Characteristics: Facial rash with "slapped face" appearance, maculopapular red spots on upper and lower extremities
- Complications: Self-limited arthritis and arthralgia
- Treatment: Symptomatic antipyretics and analgesics
- Vaccine: None available
- Nursing management: Isolation is not necessary except in child with immunosuppression and aplastic crises

ROSEOLA (EXANTHEMA SUBITUM)

- Transmission: Unknown but limited to children 6 months to 3 years
- Characteristics: High fever in child who looks well; rose-pink macules on trunk that spread to neck, face, and extremities; nonpruritic, cervical, and postauricular lymphadenopathy; inflamed pharynx; cough; coryza
- Complications: Recurrent febrile seizures and, rarely, encephalitis
- Treatment: Nonspecific, antipyretics for fever
- Vaccine: None available
- Nursing management: Discuss precautions if child is prone to febrile seizures

MEASLES (RUBEOLA)

- Transmission: Respiratory droplet spread; direct contact with respiratory tract secretions, blood, or urine
- Characteristics: Fever, malaise, cough, conjunctivitis, photophobia, Koplik spots, red rash on face that spreads downward, anorexia, lymphadenopathy, and desquamation
- Complications: Otitis, pneumonia, bronchiolitis, obstructive laryngitis, encephalitis
- Treatment: Supportive care
- Vaccine: Available; see the Center for Disease Control and Prevention's Web site, www.cdc.gov/vaccines
- Nursing management: Respiratory isolation until 5th day of rash, antipyretics, dim lights for photophobia, examine cornea for signs of ulceration, vaporizer, tepid baths

MUMPS

- Transmission: Direct contact or airborne via droplet
- Characteristics: Fever, headache, anorexia followed by earache, swollen parotid gland(s) accompanied by pain and tenderness
- Complications: Sensorineural deafness, postinfectious encephalitis, myocarditis, arthritis, hepatitis, sterility (rare in men), meningitis, epididymo-orchitis
- Treatment: Analgesics, antipyretics, fluids
- Vaccine: Available; see the Center for Disease Control and Prevention's Web site, www.cdc.gov/vaccines
- Nursing management: Isolation, analgesics, antipyretics, fluids, and hot or cold packs to neck; for orchitis, support with tight-fitting underwear

PERTUSSIS OR WHOOPING COUGH (BORDETELLA PERTUSSIS)

- Transmission: Direct contact or droplet spread from infected person
- Characteristics: Upper respiratory infection (URI) symptoms for 1–2 weeks, followed by severe hacking cough (paroxysmal stage), sneezing, low-grade fever. Coughing is more frequent at night, associated with high-pitched crowing or whoop that lasts 4–6 weeks.
- Complications: Atelectasis, otitis media, pneumonia, seizures, weight loss, hernia, prolapsed rectum
- Treatment: Azithromycin, pertussis immunoglobulin
- Vaccine: Available; see the Center for Disease Control and Prevention's Web site, www.cdc.gov/vaccines
- Nursing management: Isolation, bedrest, and hospitalization may be required for infants and dehydrated children; assess respiratory function for possible intubation; have oxygen available; encourage fluids; use high humidity

POLIOMYELITIS (ENTEROVIRUSES)

- Transmission: Direct contact with infected person via fecal-oral and pharyngeal-oropharyngeal routes
- Characteristics are in three forms:
  - Fever, sore throat, headache, anorexia, vomiting, abdominal pain lasting hours to days
  - All previous symptoms with pain and stiff neck, back, and legs
  - Same as above with recovery, then signs of CNS paralysis
- Complications: Permanent paralysis, respiratory arrest, hypertension, kidney stones from demineralization of bones during immobility
- Treatment: Respiratory assistance for respiratory paralysis, physical therapy after acute phase
- Vaccine: Available; see the Center for Disease Control and Prevention's Web site, www.cdc.gov/vaccines
- Nursing management: Maintain complete bedrest during acute phase, administer mild sedatives, use moist hot packs, range of motion (ROM) exercise, observe for respiratory paralysis

GERMAN MEASLES (RUBELLA)

- Transmission: Nasopharyngeal secretions, blood, stool, and urine
- Characteristics: Low-grade fever, headache, malaise, lymphadenopathy, sore throat, and then rash; rash on face spreads downward in red-pink maculopapular exanthema that disappears by day 3
- Complications: Teratogenic effects on fetus; condition may lead to arthritis, encephalitis, or purpura (rare)
- Treatment: Antipyretics for fever
- Vaccine: MMR available; see the Center for Disease Control and Prevention's Web site, www.cdc.gov/vaccines
- Nursing management includes isolating client from pregnant women

SCARLET FEVER (GROUP A ß-HEMOLYTIC STREPTOCOCCI)
- Transmission: Direct contact, droplet spread, or contact with articles contaminated with Group A ß-hemolytic streptococci
- Characteristics: Abrupt high fever, vomiting, headache, chills, malaise, abdominal pain, enlarged tonsils
- Complications: Peritonsillar and retropharyngeal abscess, sinusitis, glomerulonephritis, carditis, polyarthritis
- Treatment: Penicillin or erythromycin
- Vaccine: Available; see the Center for Disease Control and Prevention's Web site, www.cdc.gov/vaccines
- Nursing management: Respiratory precautions until 24 hours after start of antibiotics

Middle Childhood

IMPETIGO (*STAPHYLOCOCCUS*)
- Transmission: Auto-innocular and contagious by contact
- Characteristics: Reddish macule that becomes vesicular, ruptures easily leaving moist erosion, sharply marginated irregular outlines; exudates form honey-colored crusts; pruritus
- Complications: Secondary infections
- Treatment: Topical bactericidal ointment; oral or parenteral antibiotics (penicillin) when severe
- Nursing management: Careful removal of crusts, comfort care

SCABIES (INFESTATION WITH SCABIES MITE, *SARCOPTES SCABIEI*)
- Transmission: Prolonged contact with the mite: it requires about 45 minutes for the mite to burrow under the skin
- Characteristics: Intense itching, which may lead to excoriations secondary to scratching; maculopapular lesions occur interdigitally and in axillary, popliteal, and inguinal areas
- Complications: Secondary infections
- Treatment: Application of a scabicide such as Elimite; persons in close proximity to an infested person should be treated
- Nursing management: Educate families about accurately following directions for use of scabicide; elimite should be applied to all skin surfaces, with care to avoid eye contact; touching and holding child should be minimized and nurses should wear gloves

LICE (*PEDICULOSIS CAPITIS*)
- Transmission: Person to person or sharing of personal items
- Characteristics: Scalp itching and irritation
- Complications: Scratch marks and inflammatory papules caused by secondary infections
- Treatment: Application of pediculicides (Nix or RID) and manual removal of nits; daily removal of nits should continue until no longer found
- Nursing management: Educate families that anyone can get lice; lice do not jump or fly and are not transmitted by pets; lice survive for 48 hours away from the host, but nits are shed into the environment and can hatch in 7–10 days

LYME DISEASE (SPIROCHETE *BORRELIA BURGDORFERI*)
- Transmission: Tick bite, especially the deer tick
- Characteristics in Stage 1: Erythema chronicum migrans at bite with raised doughnut-like border, pain described as burning, warm to touch, occasionally pruritic; fever, headache, malaise, anorexia, stiff neck, generalized lymphadenopathy, splenomegaly, sore throat, conjunctivitis, cough
- Complications in Stage 2: Neurologic, cardiac, and musculoskeletal involvement 2–11 weeks after cutaneous symptoms
- Complications in Stage 3: Musculoskeletal pains occur months or years later; chronic arthritis; late neurological problems may include deafness, encephalopathy, and keratitis
- Treatment: Amoxicillin or penicillin <8 years old; doxycycline or amoxicillin ≥8 years old; cefuroxime and erythromycin if allergic
- Vaccine: None available
- Nursing management: Education to protect from tick exposure through avoidance, use of repellent such as DEET (diethyltoluamide) or permethrin for children >1 year old

CAT SCRATCH DISEASE
- A common regional lymphadenitis in children and teens; benign and self-limited, resolves spontaneously in 2–4 months
- Transmission: 90% of the time follows scratch or bite of an animal leading to infection with *Bartonella henselae*, gram-negative bacteria
- Characteristics: Erythematous papule at inoculation—painless and nonpruritic
- Complications: Encephalitis, hepatitis
- Treatment: Supportive care
- Vaccine: None available
- Nursing management: Limit activity to prevent trauma to enlarged lymph nodes, bedrest for those with fever, analgesics for discomfort, but there is no need to get rid of pet

Adolescence
ACNE VULGARIS
- Increased sebum production causing inflamed papules, pustules, nodules, and cysts; begins in early adolescence and gradually increases until late teens
- Characteristics: Formation of blackheads (open comedones) or whiteheads (closed comedones); proliferation of *P. acnes*, a benign organism always present on the skin
- Complications: Secondary infection, scarring
- Treatment: Supportive care and specific treatments determined by type of lesions; resolves slowly over 6+ weeks; topical benzoyl peroxide inhibits bacterial growth; Accutane may be used in severe cases, but pregnancy must be prevented when using this medication
- Nursing management: Explanation of disease process, education about gentle cleansing

TRACTION

The purpose of traction is immobilization to maintain proper alignment of fractures.

Types
- Skin traction: Pull is applied to skin and indirectly to skeletal structures.
- Skeletal traction: Pull is applied directly to bone by pins, wires, or tongs through the diameter of the bone.
- External fixators: Portable devices attached by percutaneous pins or wires to the leg bone for correction of deformities, limb lengthening, or pseudoarthroses.
- Bryant traction: Running traction in which the pull is in one direction only. The legs are flexed at 90° angle at the hips and the buttocks are raised slightly off the bed, resulting in countertraction.
- Buck extension: Used for short-term immobilization (e.g., for dislocation, Legg-Calvé-Perthes); the legs are extended.
- Russell traction: Skin traction applied to lower leg with padded sling under the knee, creating two lines of pull (longitudinal and perpendicular) and allowing some position changes without malalignment.
- Cervical traction: Helps prevent dislocation or fracture of the vertebrae which may result in spinal cord injury (Halo; Crutchfield, Barton, or Gardner-Wells tongs).

Care of Child With Traction
- Ensure equipment is properly positioned with correct amount of weight, weights freely hanging, pulleys correctly aligned, body in alignment.
- Assess skin under straps and pin insertion sites for redness, edema, skin breakdown, and drainage.
- Assess extremity for neurovascular status.
- Monitor for pain and skin condition of prominences lying on bed.
- Sterile pin care.
- Provide skin care every 4 hours, using sheepskin under affected extremity.

PHARMACOLOGY

Growth and maturation of children contribute to the body's capacity to metabolize and excrete medications. Immaturity of organs, or problems with absorption, distribution, metabolism, or excretion, can significantly alter effects of medications. Newborn and premature babies with immature enzyme systems in the liver are particularly vulnerable to harmful effects of drugs.

Drug Interactions
Nurses and parents need to be aware of possible drug interactions, particularly with antihistamines. One example is the use of astemizole (Hismanal), which, if given with erythromycin, can lead to life-threatening cardiac dysrhythmias. Stevens-Johnson syndrome (erythema multiforme), sometimes associated with ingestion of drugs used for upper-respiratory infection, manifests as a rash and lesions and has a morality rate of about 10%.

- *Over-the-counter:* Concern over the use of antihistamines, decongestants, antitussives, and expectorants has been growing among pediatricians. Pharmaceutical companies continue to market the drugs for children, but the efficacy is not well-documented and should not be given to any child under the age of 2 years (Sharfstein, North, & Serwint, 2007).
- *Herbal:* In recent years investigators have reported widespread use of alternative medicines. Some herbal therapies have potentially harmful side effects as well as adverse interactions with medications. It is therefore important for healthcare providers to have knowledge about herbal medications, to inquire about their use, and to educate families about the risks and benefits, as well as potential interactions these products may have with over-the-counter and prescription medications (Lanski, Greenwalk, Perkins, & Simon, 2003).
- *Complementary and alternative medicine (CAM)* includes a variety of products and practices not currently a part of conventional medicine. They are primarily used for chronic medical conditions, and evidence to determine safety and effectiveness is ongoing. There are five classes of therapy:
  - Biologically based: Foods, diets, vitamins, herbal, or plant preparations
  - Manipulative treatment: Chiropractic, osteopathy, massage
  - Energy-based: Reiki, magnetic treatment, pulsed fields current
  - Mind-body techniques: Mental healing, relaxation, hypnosis, expressive
  - Alternative medical systems: Homeopathy, naturopathy, ayurvedic, traditional Chinese medicine, including acupuncture and moxicombustion (Hockenberry & Wilson, 2009).

Prescription

After a drug is prescribed to a child, careful diligence is needed to determine the correct dose, watching for side effects or complications. Antiarrhythmics, anticoagulants, chemotherapeutic agents, electrolytes, and insulin should be double-checked by another nurse prior to being administered to a child; they may be hazardous or even lethal at incorrect doses.

- *Therapeutic drug levels* need to be monitored because children respond to drugs so differently. Evaluation of side effects and toxic effects is also useful to determine correct dosages.
- *Weight-specific dosing* has been used to determine safe doses for children. Most often the method used is mg/kg. The most reliable method is to calculate the body surface area (BSA), using a nomogram derived from the height and weight of a child.

Total Parenteral Nutrition (TPN)

TPN is also known as IV alimentation or hyperalimentation and provides for the nutritional needs of infants or children. Total nutrient admixture (TNA) may refer to 1) minerals, water, trace elements, and other additives in a single container; or 2) dextrose, amino acids, and lipids in a single solution. TPN often refers to dextrose and amino acids with additives to which lipids are piggybacked into the system.

Indications for Use
- Include chronic intestinal obstruction or conditions preventing bowel function, malabsorption, severe diarrhea, or extensive body burn.

Requirements
- For infusion, include use of a large vessel such as superior vena cava, innominate vein, or internal jugular vein to minimize phlebitis and irritation.

Caveats
- Use strict aseptic technique to prevent bacterial growth with high-glucose, high-protein solutions.
- Avoid adding other solutions or medicines in the line.

Complications
- Liver disease, especially in preterm infants.
- Imbalance in elements, such as hypoglycemia.
- Catheter-related events, such as infection, sepsis, venous thrombosis, embolization, and/or endocarditis.

Nursing Actions
- Monitor for blood sugar changes.
- Allow infants to suck nonnutritively to fulfill oral needs.
- Monitor for liver changes.
- Reassess requirements for growth.
- Monitor social and motor development because IV infusion may reduce mobility and socialization.

NUTRITION

Early eating habits are especially important in developing healthy children. Nutrition is often regarded as the most important determinant of growth. The nurse can be instrumental in guiding parents in food selection for their children. During early childhood, a child is growing rapidly with an associated demand for calories, particularly protein. There are many plateaus and growth spurts, and a child's nutritive needs may change, but habits are developed early and care should be taken to ensure those are healthy habits.

Nutrition Guidelines
Nutritional assessment can be completed through careful clinical exams, evaluating hair, skin, and mouth particularly. In addition, diet intakes can be used, but may be inaccurate. Finally, biochemical analysis helps inform adequate nutrition.

Routes
While oral feedings are the most satisfying to young children, they also may be fed by nasogastric tube or intravenously.

Formulas
Breastfeeding or formula is recommended during the first year of life because of infants' inability to tolerate cow's milk. For the first 6 months, human milk is the most desirable and complete diet. Even though breast milk is relatively low in iron, it is absorbed better than iron-fortified formula. Additional iron (400 IU daily) may be added if a mother's iron intake is inadequate. Addition of solid foods may begin at 4–6 months and should be added one food at a time. Rice cereal is generally the first food introduced to an infant. Tooth eruption begins at about 6 months of age. Finger foods such as crackers, raw fruit, or vegetables can be added.

Vitamins/Supplements

Necessary for specific metabolic activity, vitamins are an essential food element and important in growth and development. A deficiency of a vitamin can affect metabolic activity, and excessive amounts of vitamins may have a toxic effect on a child because of organ immaturity. As long as a child maintains a balanced diet in adequate amounts, vitamin deficiencies are rare in the United States. Fat-soluble vitamins (A, D, E, and K) are found in many foods and stored in the liver. Vitamin K is also synthesized by intestinal bacteria and vitamin D becomes available to the body through exposure to sunlight.

Therapeutic/Alternative Diets

Vegetarians and alternative diets are becoming more common and care must be taken to ensure children maintain adequate nutrition while excluding meat and other foods from their diets. Various types of diets include:

- Lacto-ovo-vegetarians exclude animal flesh but eat dairy products and eggs
- Lacto-vegetarians exclude animal flesh and eggs but eat dairy products
- Vegans exclude animal flesh, dairy products, and eggs
- Zen macrobiotics exclude meat, poultry, milk, and eggs, and eat large amounts of leafy, root, and sea vegetables, and fruit and fish
- Semi-vegetarians are lacto-ovo-vegetarian, but eat poultry and fish (Hockenberry & Wilson, 2009)

Growth Charts

An important aspect of a child's physical exam is growth in relationship to previous growth patterns and in relationship to other children's growth. The National Center for Health Statistics has revised growth charts to include BMI, heights, weights, and head circumferences for ages birth–20 years. Three important indicators for further evaluation are:

- Widely disparate height and weight percentiles
- Failure to show expected growth rates
- Sudden increase or decrease in previously steady growth (except in puberty)

BMI

Body mass index is equal to [weight in pounds/height in inches/height in inches] x 703. This measurement represents the relationship between height and weight. It can be either calculated or found on a nomogram. A child is described as overweight if she or he falls above the 85th percentile. The BMI is helpful in detecting early signs of risk for being overweight and obesity. The prevalence of being overweight and obesity among children has greatly increased over the past decade (Hedley, Ogden, Johnson, Carroll, Curtin, & Flegal, 2004). The most prevalent physical complication of childhood obesity is diabetes. However, self-esteem and psychosocial problems also may occur. Obesity may persist into adulthood with the additional risks of heart disease and joint problems.

CHEMISTRY

Body Fluid Balance/Imbalance

Infants and young children are more susceptible to fluid and electrolyte imbalance because it develops rapidly in children and they adjust less quickly. Children tend to run higher fevers than adults because of:

- Increased surface area (skin) relative to size: preemie has 5x, infant has 2–3x body surface area/kg compared to an adult
- Higher metabolic rate
- Immature kidney of infant doesn't concentrate or dilute urine, conserve or excrete sodium, or acidify urine

Children may experience dehydration, water intoxication, or edema.

- Dehydration is classified as isotonic, hypotonic, or hypertonic. The most common causes of dehydration are loss of fluid from vomiting, diarrhea, diabetic ketoacidosis, and extensive burns.

Electrolyte Balance/Imbalance

- Hyponatremia occurs with loss of sodium (Na) through sweating, replaced with water, resulting in weakness, dizziness, nausea, apathy, weak pulse, decreased blood pressure, lethargy, Na <130.
- Hypernatremia results in intense thirst; dry, sticky mucous membranes; flushed skin; oliguria; nausea; hoarseness; increased temperature; Na >150.
- Hypokalemia (low serum potassium [K]) manifests as muscle weakness, cramping, hypotension, cardiac arrhythmias, ileus, tachy- or bradycardia, irritability, apathy or drowsiness, fatigue, K <3.5.
- Hyperkalemia can result in hyperreflexia, twitching, muscle weakness, flaccid paralysis, bradycardia, ventricular fibrillation and arrest, oliguria, apnea and arrest, K ≥5.5.
- Hypocalcemia manifests as tingling of nose, ears, toes, fingers; tetany, convulsions, laryngospasm, neuromuscular irritability; hypotension, cardiac arrest; Ca <8.5 mg/dL.
- Hypercalcemia results in constipation, weakness, fatigue, nausea, anorexia, thirst, bradycardia or arrest, increased calcium in urine causing kidney stones, muscle hypotonicity.

Clinical Signs Associated With Isotonic Dehydration in Infants

- Children with isotonic dehydration typically display symptoms of hypovolemic shock (Hockenberry & Wilson, 2009), reduced size of vascular compartment
- Falling blood pressure
- Low central venous pressure
- Poor capillary filling

Clinical Observations Important With Fluid Balance
- Intake and output
- Heart rate—tachycardia
- Temperature—elevated
- Respirations—rapid
- Blood pressure—children compensate so decreased BP is critical
- Skin color, turgor, temperature, elasticity

- Edema
- Mucous membranes
- Fontanel
- Salivation and tearing
- Eyeballs
- Muscle cramps
- Behavior
- Weight
- Urine output—should be at least 1cc/kg/hr

Acid–Base Balance

Disturbances in acid–base balance include respiratory acidosis, respiratory alkalosis, metabolic acidosis, and metabolic alkalosis.

NORMAL LABORATORY VALUES
- pH: 7.35–7.45
- pO_2: 80–100
- pCO_2: 35–45
- HCO_3: 22–26
- Electrolytes
  - K: 3.5–5.0 mEq/L
  - Na: 136–149 mEq/L
  - Cl: 98–106 mEq/L

REFERENCES

Hedley, A. A., Ogden, C. L., Johnson, C. L., Carroll, M. D., Curtin, L. R., & Flegal, K. M. (2004). Prevalence of overweight and obesity among U.S. children, adolescents, and adults, 1999–2002. *JAMA, 291*, 2847–2850.

Hockenberry, M. J., & Wilson, D. (2009). *Wong's nursing care of infants and children* (8th ed.). St. Louis, MO: Mosby Elsevier.

Kuczmarski, R. J. (2000). *CDC growth charts: United States. Advance data from vital and health statistics.* Retrieved from http://www.cdc.gov/growthcharts/

Lanski, S. T., Greenwald, M., Perkins, A., & Simon, H. (2003). Herbal therapy use in a pediatric emergency department population: Expect the unexpected. *Pediatrics, 111*, 981–985.

London, M. L., Ladewig P. W., Ball, J. W., & Bindler, R. C. (2007). *Maternal and child nursing care* (2nd ed.). Upper Saddle River, NJ: Pearson Prentice Hall.

Sharfstein, J. M., North, M., & Serwint, J. R. (2007). Over the counter but no longer under the radar. *NEJM, 357*, 2321–2324.

6

Educational Principles and Strategies

Karen Corlett, MSN, RN-BC, CPNP-AC/PC, PNP-BC

This chapter is meant as a framework to describe the process and components of patient and family teaching that is undertaken by nurses on a daily basis. The actual content of patient and family education will be discussed in the sections devoted to the major health problems.

PATIENT EDUCATION

- Begins at first contact
  - Emergency department
  - Preoperative visit
  - Admission
  - Well-child visit
  - Clinic visit
- Necessary for health promotion and disease prevention
- Important in management of acute and chronic disease
  - Increasing importance as more care is undertaken in the home

Preprocedure Teaching

Assessment of Learning Needs
- Age, developmental stage
  - Affects timing of preparation, depth of information, and word choices
- Background
  - Past history and experience with healthcare system
  - Culture, religion
  - Family attitudes and family dynamics
  - Previous information supplied
- Current knowledge and expectations

Planning and Delivery of Patient Education
- Encourage participation of child
- Encourage parental involvement
  - May have different personnel or physical spaces to meet developmental and educational needs of both child and caregivers
- Developmentally appropriate play as learning tool
  - Coloring, painting
  - Dolls, toys
  - Medical play with safe medical equipment
  - Familiarize child with the environment

Reinforcement of Learning
- Through daily activities, nursing care, and play activities
- Support parents/family in their ability to reinforce education

Evaluation of Learning
- Ask child to explain plan of care or upcoming tests/procedures
- Correct and reinforce as indicated

Patient/Family Teaching as One Component of the Education Process

Assessment of Learning Needs
- Prioritized objectives
  - Need to know vs. nice to know
  - Consider time available and attention span

Assessment of Barriers to Learning
- For patient
- For family or other caregivers

Planning and Delivery of Patient Education
- Teaching methods based on preference and abilities of learner
  - Verbal information
  - Printed materials: flyers, posters, books, articles
  - Audio and/or video presentations

    – Interactive audio/video presentations
    – Demonstration
       • Simulations
       • Return demonstration of learned skills
    – Individual vs. group learning environment

Reinforcement of Education
* Targeted to priority knowledge and skills
* Positive feedback for gained skill/knowledge
* Constructive correction where indicated

Evaluation of Learning
* Pre-/posttest comparisons
* Recitation of knowledge
* Return demonstration of skills
    – Simulations
    – Actual performance

Revision of Teaching Methods, Plan, Target Knowledge
* Based on evaluation of learning
    – Input from teacher and learner(s)
* Implementation of revised plan

Barriers to Effective Learning
* Lack of readiness for change or learning
    – Acceptance of illness or deficit is necessary before being motivated to take care of new needs
* Differences in health beliefs or practice
* Visual, cognitive, auditory, language, or learning disabilities or deficits
* Use of healthcare jargon
* Anxiety, drug or disease effects, environmental distractions
* Culturally insensitive teaching
* Developmental stage or educational abilities of the learner not taken into account
    – Consider regression of developmental maturity and limited learning abilities in times of stress or illness
* Organizational barriers to effective patient/family education
    – Space, noise, privacy, time, and resource constraints

Support in Place to Continue Necessary Learning
* Community resources and support
* Disease management or lifestyle change specific resources and support
    – Leukemia and Lymphoma Society
    – Juvenile Diabetes Association
    – National Organization of Rare Diseases
    – Cystic Fibrosis Foundation

REFERENCES

Chamberlain, R. S. (2005). Care of the sick or hospitalized child. In E. J. Mills (Ed.), *Lippincott manual of nursing practice* (8th ed., pp. 1382–1422). Philadelphia: Lippincott Williams & Wilkins.

Donaldson, N. E., Rutledge, D. N., & Pravikoff, D. S. (2000). *Principles of effective adult-focused patient education in nursing.* Glendale, CA: Cinahl Information Systems.

Potts, N. L., & Mandleco, B. L. (Eds.). (2007). *Pediatric nursing: Caring for children and their families* (2nd ed.). Clifton Park, NY: Tomson.

Russell, S. S. (2006). An overview of adult-learning processes. *Urologic Nursing, 26*(5), 349–352, 370.

7

Life Situations and Adaptive/ Maladaptive Responses

Karen Corlett, MSN, RN-BC, CPNP-AC/PC, PNP-BC

END-OF-LIFE CARE

- Physical care and emotional support of the dying child and grieving family

Understanding the Concept of Death
Age-Appropriate Explanations
- Young children do not understand death as permanent
- School-age children understand that death is final and not reversible
  - Understand concept of death but typically can't envision their own
- Older children begin to understand that everyone must die
- Teenagers see themselves as invincible
  - Experiencing death of peer shakes this core belief
- Children and teens begin to associate death with causality
  - Accuracy of this correlation depends on developmental stage
- Previous experiences with death or dying influence understanding

Education in Child-Friendly Manner
- Developmentally targeted books, stories, role play
  - Child life, social work, chaplain, psychiatry departments can be helpful
  - Can also help parents and caregivers with developmentally appropriate explanations for children
- Sensitivity to parents' desires regarding cultural or religious philosophies

Family Education
- Process of death
  - Assistance with physical care needs
  - Developmentally appropriate explanations of physical symptoms and activity changes associated with the dying process
- Impact of death on family unit, siblings
- Grief support
  - In anticipation of death
  - Once death occurs
    - Community resources

Stages of Grief (Kübler-Ross)
Denial
- Denial of risk of death or actual death

Anger
- Why me, why my child

Bargaining
- Desire to trade places with the dying child
- Bargaining to live until a certain time, holiday, or special event

Depression
- Not wanting to go on
- Not caring about life, grieving parent not caring about remaining family

Acceptance
- Of death or probability of death

Palliative Care
- Care for those with chronic conditions for which there is no cure
  - Does not need to be imminent risk of death
  - Often a team approach
    - Physician, nursing, social work, psychiatry, pain management, pharmacy, nutrition, child life, and others may be represented on team
- Can begin at any time from diagnosis to near end of life
  - Ideally begun early in course of disease
- Assist with care and planning for best possible life despite potential limitations of disease
  - Does not imply limitation of care or limitation of resuscitation
  - Care choices emphasize symptom management, including comfort and function

- Patients/families may cycle in and out of aggressive vs. comfort care during the course of their disease
- Palliative care can coexist with hospice care toward end of life

RESPONSE TO CRISIS

Diagnosis or Hospitalization
- Kübler-Ross's stages of grief

Response of Patient
- Dependent on age and developmental stage
- Understanding of disease process and outcomes
- Change from usual routines
  PHYSIOLOGIC
  - Nutrition, sleep, pain

  PSYCHOLOGIC AND ENVIRONMENTAL
  - Few familiar/comforting objects or people
  - Pain
  - Change in daily routine
  - Inability to be held/comforted in usual manner
  - Separation from family and peers
    - Promote family-centered care

Response of Family
- Change in family unit
  - Patient's role in family prior to illness

  CHANGE IN FAMILY MEMBERS' ROLES DUE TO ILLNESS
  - Breadwinner to caregiver
  - Stay-at-home parent to hospital caregiver
  - Sibling becomes caregiver or household manager in absence of stay-at-home parent
  - Grandparent becomes primary caregiver of well siblings
  - Neighbor to chauffeur of well siblings or for patient

  TEMPORARY VS. PERMANENT ADJUSTMENT TO NEW ROLES
  - May be difficult for some to flex in and out of roles as needs wax and wane
  - May be difficult transition to new or old role once crisis is resolved

The Vulnerable Child Syndrome
Parental Perception That the Child Is at Higher Risk of Illness, Injury, or Death
- After full recovery from a perceived or actual life-threatening illness
- Difficult conception, pregnancy, or birth
- When the child reminds the parent of someone who experienced premature death

Parent Behaviors Toward the "Vulnerable Child"
- Treating the child as younger than chronologic or developmental age
- Difficulty with discipline and limit-setting
- Overindulgent or overcontrolling parenting
- Excessive concern about child's health/wellness and frequent visits to healthcare providers
- Difficulty separating from child

Nursing Management
- Gather data regarding child/family risks for vulnerable child syndrome
  - Ask about previous serious illness (real or perceived)
  - Ask about parental fears for child
  - Observe parenting behaviors
- Assess for presence of risk factors for vulnerable child syndrome
- Parental awareness of issues may bring change in behavior
- Family counseling for those with continued parenting difficulties

Coping Mechanisms
- Behaviors that attempt to decrease stress

Action-Oriented Behaviors
- Planning
- Learning
- Limiting competing activities
  - Preserving energy for the stressor
- Restraint or self-control
- Confrontation
- The problem causing the stress is addressed, improved, or eliminated

Emotion-Based Behaviors: Can Be Adaptive or Maladaptive Depending Upon Situation and Frequency
- Denial
- Avoidance
- Sleep or relaxation
- Hope, positive thinking
- Repression
- Distraction
- Humor

Maladaptive Responses
Suicide or Suicidal Ideation
- Teens have highest incidence
  - RISKS AND WARNING SIGNS
    - Major life stressor
    - Depression
    - Talk of suicide
    - Suicide event in community
    - Giving away possessions or making a will

- School failure
- Mood swings
- Loss of interest in food, personal appearance, relationships

ASSESSMENT OF LETHALITY AND RISK
- Does the child have a plan
  - Time, method, access to method
  - Rescue opportunity in place
    - Remote location for event vs. knowing parent will arrive home shortly after swallowing pills
- Referral for protective custody if danger to self or others

Substance Abuse
- Alcohol, tobacco, prescription, over-the-counter or illicit drugs
  WARNING SIGNS
  - Change in habits
    - Hygiene, appearance, food preferences, appetite
  - Change in mood
  - School failure
  - Change in peer group
  - Smell of drugs or alcohol
    - Finding drugs, alcohol, or paraphernalia of use
  - Illegal acts

Depression
MAY BE SITUATIONALLY APPROPRIATE DEPRESSION OF MOOD
- Limited duration
- Return to full functionality

CLINICAL DEPRESSION
- Refer for professional care and counseling
- Entire family may need to be part of counseling

SIGNS AND SYMPTOMS OF DEPRESSION
- Depressed mood
- Inability to enjoy usual activities
- Weight gain or loss
- Difficulty concentrating
- Insomnia or hypersomnia
- Lack of self-worth
- Thoughts of, or attempts at, suicide
- Change in family or peer relationships
- Change in school performance
- Change in appearance, clothing, hygiene

ASSESSMENT
- Reliable tools for measurements of childhood depression
- Children's Depression Inventory
- Children's Depression Rating Scale

Posttraumatic Stress Disorder
ANXIETY DISORDER FOLLOWING A LIFE-THREATENING OR TRAUMATIC EVENT
- Natural disasters
- Accidents
- Conflict incidents
  - War, murder, abuse, rape
- Symptoms
  - Reexperiencing the trauma or event
    · Dreams, intrusive thoughts
    · May be expressed in child's play
  - Avoidance of situation that triggers memories of event
    · Avoidance of feelings related to event
    · Numbing of feelings
    · Lack of enjoyment
  - Hypervigilance
    · Startles easily
    · Difficulty sleeping
- Nursing care
  - Referral for specialty care
  - Build trusting relationship
  - Explore trauma and meaning
    · Validate child's experience of and reaction to traumatic event
    · Lift responsibility for event from child
  - Increase coping repertoire

Eating Disorders
COMPLEX SET OF BEHAVIORS RELATED TO FOOD
- Multifactorial causation
- Most common in teens but age at onset decreasing
- Girls > boys

ANOREXIA NERVOSA
- Severe food restriction
- Altered body image
- Weight loss
  - Irrational fear of weight gain and/or becoming fat
- Underweight
- Physical manifestations of weight loss
  - Hypothermia and cold intolerance
  - Hair loss and brittle nails
    · May grow fine hair on body (lanugo)
  - Skipping or stopping of menstrual cycles
  - Cardiac dysrhythmia
- Significant morbidity and mortality
  - Fluid and electrolyte abnormalities can be life threatening

BULIMIA
- Cycle of binging (excessive calorie intake) and subsequent purging
  - Laxative use
  - Induced vomiting
  - Excessive exercise
  - Fasting
- Feeling of lack of control over food
- Underweight not required for diagnosis

PSYCHOLOGICAL DIAGNOSES
- DSM criteria for diagnosis
- Require ongoing treatment of patient and family

Child Maltreatment

INTENTIONAL INJURY OF A CHILD
- 1,460 reported child deaths from abuse in 2005
- An underreported statistic

CHILD NEGLECT
- Lack of provision for physical, emotional, or educational needs
  - Nutrition, health care, safe environment, school attendance
  - Due to intentional abuse, neglect, or lack of knowledge
- Chronic neglect
  - Lack of clean environment, inadequate nutrition
- Acute neglect resulting in injury (e.g., lack of supervision around a pool, bathtub, lake, or river resulting in a drowning)

PHYSICAL ABUSE
- Results in bodily injury
  - Bruises, bites, burns, broken bones, brain injury

EMOTIONAL ABUSE
- Lack of affection or emotional support
- Continued belittling of the child
- Can affect physical growth and development in addition to emotional growth and maturation
- All forms of abuse have emotional effects on the child

SEXUAL ABUSE
- Inappropriate touching or sexual behavior between an adult and a child

MOST PERPETRATORS OF ABUSE ARE CAREGIVERS
- Relatives next most common
- Nonrelatives in position of authority
  - Coach, minister, teacher, group leader, and so on
- Strangers are rarest of perpetrators

CHILDREN AT RISK
- The very young
  - Children <3 years old have highest rates of abuse
  - Most dependent, neglect highest in this age group
- General risks
  - Stress events
  - Living below the poverty level
  - Caretaker has experienced abuse or violence
  - Caretaker with limited coping strategies for stress
  - Caregiver depression

INJURIES THAT SHOULD RAISE CONCERN ABOUT ABUSE
- Any injury not consistent with the reported story
  - Discrepancies in story
  - Repeated injuries
- Fractures
  - Ribs, scapula, sternum, or metacarpals
- Burns
  - Multiple healed or healing burns
  - Immersion burns
    - Flexor areas spared as child tries to protect self from hot liquid
  - Contact burns
    - May have shape of identifiable object (cigarette, curling iron, brand, and so on)
- Shaken baby syndrome
  - Subdural hematoma
  - Retinal injury
  - Rib or other occult bone fractures
  - Caused by vigorous shaking of the child
    - Child's large head for size causes coup-countercoup injury and shear injury to blood vessels and brain tissue
  - One-third of affected children die, one-third have serious residual injury from the shaking
- Munchausen syndrome by proxy
  - Psychological disorder of the parent
    - Parent creates illness in child
    - Parent gains positive experience from interaction with healthcare professionals
    - Parent often has some type of healthcare background
    - Parent may go to elaborate measures to continue the symptoms/ appearance of chronic illness in the child
    - Child may become technology-dependent due to parental claims of symptoms
    - Difficult to diagnose, symptoms often subjective (apnea, feeding intolerance, seizures are common complaints)
    - As with most cases of abuse, child will protect the parent

NURSES ARE MANDATORY REPORTERS
- MUST report documented or suspected child maltreatment to authorities
- Can be reported by another discipline in the institution such as social work
  - Reports can be anonymous
  - Reports must be investigated by state agency

PREVENTION
- Education
  - Nationally, locally, and individually
  - Prenatal and postnatal education
  - Stress management
  - Community services and resources
- In-home support
  - By nurses, social workers, or other agency representatives
  - Education, evaluation, and connection to community resources
- Regular visits to healthcare provider
  - Physical exam
  - Psychosocial assessment
    · Coping repertoires
    · Depression or other psychological disorders
    · Respite opportunities
- Out-of-home child care
  - As respite for continuous child care responsibilities
  - Model for child of healthy interactions
- Life skills training
  - For new parents
  - For older children who have experienced abuse
- Family support services
  - Community agencies
  - Facilitating personal support networks
- Public education
  - Awareness of problem
  - Risk factors to be aware of
  - Ways to support those at risk
  - Solicitation of financial support for agencies

REFERENCES

Cohn Donnelly, A. (1997). *An approach to preventing child abuse.* Retrieved from http://member.
preventchildabuse.org/site/DocServer/an_approach_to_prevention.pdf?docID=121

Kübler-Ross, E., & Kessler, D. (2005). *On grief and grieving: Finding the meaning of grief through the
five stages of loss.* New York: Simon & Schuster Ltd.

U.S. Department of Health and Human Services, Children's Bureau. (2007). *Child maltreatment 2005.*
Retrieved from http://www.acf.hhs.gov/programs/cb/pubs/cm05/index.htm

8

Sensory Disorders

Clara J. Richardson, MSN, RN-BC

HEARING DISORDERS

Description

Hearing disorders in children are defined as hard of hearing: loss of 25–70 dBHL (decibel hearing level); and as deaf: loss of more than 70 dBHL. The loss may be unilateral or bilateral.

Etiology

A conductive hearing loss is due to dysfunction of the external or middle ear. Sensorineural loss is caused by impairment of the cochlea or auditory nerve. A mixed loss has both sensory and conductive components.

Causes of conductive loss are malformation of the outer or middle ear and, more often, infections of the middle ear. Sensorineural loss is caused by hereditary factors in about half of cases. Other causes include infections, anoxic brain injury, physical trauma, prematurity, excessively loud noises, or ototoxic medications.

Incidence and Demographics

The incidence of permanent bilateral hearing loss is 0.6–2.6 per 1,000 children. Numerous genetic syndromes are associated with hearing loss and account for about 50% of cases. Sensorineural hearing loss not associated with a syndrome is more prevalent in Ashkenazi Jews, people of northern European descent, those of Japanese descent, and people from Ghana. In the United States, hearing loss is more common in males and in Blacks.

Risk Factors

- See causes above
- Cleft palate
- Neonatal hyperbilirubinemia
- Intracranial hemorrhage
- Maternal infections during pregnancy
  - Rubella
  - Cytomegalovirus (CMV)
  - Toxoplasmosis
  - Herpes virus
  - Syphilis
- Bacterial meningitis
- Down syndrome
- Chronic otitis media with effusion
- Head injury
- Ototoxic antibiotics
  - Kanamycin (Kantrex)
  - Gentamicin (Garamycin)
  - Vancomycin (Vancocin)
  - Tobramycin (Nebcin)
- Cisplatin, Carboplatin (chemotherapy)

Prevention and Screening

- Newborn screening
- Screening of children
  - Multiple episodes of otitis media with effusion
  - Cognitive disability
  - Cleft palate

Assessment

History

- Inability to localize sound by 6 months
- Delayed consonant-vowel babbling by 7 months
- Failure to respond to verbal instructions not accompanied by gestures by 16 months
- Delayed comprehensible speech by 24 months

Physical Exam

INFANTS
- No reaction to loud noise
- Delayed developmental communication milestones

OLDER CHILDREN
- Use of gestures rather than words
- Asking for repetition
- Decreased response to verbal expression
- Avoidance of social interaction
- Confused or inattentive facial expression

DIAGNOSTIC STUDIES
- Electrophysiological testing for sensorineural loss
  - Evoked otoacoustic emissions (EOAE)
  - Screening auditory brainstem response (SBAR)
- Behavioral hearing tests to distinguish sensorineural from conductive loss
  - Behavioral observation audiometry (BOA) for infants younger than 8 months
  - Visual reinforcement audiometry (VRA) for those 8 months to $2^1/_2$ years
  - Conditional play audiometry (CPA) for children older than $2^1/_2$ years
  - Speech audiometry for those older than $2^1/_2$ years
- Tympanometry to evaluate middle ear function

Management
- Invasive: Cochlear implant surgically implanted in the inner ear

Nonpharmacologic
- Amplification with hearing aids or assistive listening devices

SPEECH–LANGUAGE THERAPY
- Oralism
- American Sign Language (ASL)
- Total communication

ASSISTIVE TECHNOLOGY
- Teletypewriter
- Telecommunication devises

STRATEGIES TO ENHANCE COMMUNICATION
- Get child's attention before speaking
- Position: close, eye level, and in front of child
- Speak clearly, at even rate, and in short sentences
- Use facial expression

Pharmacologic
- No pharmacologic management indicated

Patient/Family Education
- Disability
- Amplification options
- Communication options

Outcomes and Follow-Up
- The child will have early identification of hearing impairment.
- The child will participate in an early intervention program.
- The child will utilize amplification devices.
- The child will show increased hearing with cochlear implant.
- The child will experience optimal communication.
- The family will demonstrate strategies to enhance communication with child.
- The family will verbalize understanding of disability and treatment options.

VISION DISORDERS

Description
Vision disorders in children range from low vision (partial sight), with visual acuity better than 20/200 but worse than 20/70, to blindness, with acuity of 20/200 or worse.

Etiology
Cortical Visual Impairment (CVI) Due to Damage of the Visual Cortex in the Occipital Lobe
- Hypoxia
- Infection of the central nervous system
- Traumatic brain injury

Retinopathy of Prematurity (ROP)
- Incomplete growth of the retinal blood vessels, which is not complete until 9 months gestation
- Blood vessels grow abnormally, die, and form scar tissue
- Scar tissue can cause retinal detachment and loss of vision

Optic Nerve Hypoplasia
- Nerve is small and thin and transmits impaired information to brain
- Results in sensory nystagmus, jiggling movement of the eyes

Strabismus
- Malalignment of eyes or deviation of one eye
- Results in amblyopia, reduced visual acuity in one eye

Incidence and Demographics
One-half to two-thirds of children with developmental disabilities have a significant vision disorder. Approximately 25% of newborns weighing less than 2,500 grams will have some degree of retinopathy of prematurity.

Risk Factors
- Prematurity
- Central nervous system (CNS) infection
- Traumatic brain injury
- Eye trauma

Prevention and Screening
Prevention
- Early prenatal care
- Avoid high concentrations of oxygen in premature infants
- Rubella immunization for all children
- Safety education to prevent eye trauma
- Compliance with treatment of vision impairment

Regular Vision Screening With Age-Appropriate Screening Tool
- Assessment of normal vision parameters in infants and young children
- Acuity charts

Assessment
- History of risk factors

Physical Exam
- Infant does not fixate on face or follow objects
- Eyes wandering or nystagmus
- Eyes that gaze in one direction
- No reaction to bright light or movement of object toward eye
- Focusing only on bright light

Diagnostic Studies
- See screening section above

Management
Invasive
- No invasive management indicated

Nonpharmacologic
- Textured, sound-producing toys
- Verbal cues before touching, moving from space to space
- Orientation to environment
- Self-care education
- Optical aids to enhance vision
- Braille education
- Computer training, voice recognition software
- Books on tape

Pharmacologic
- No pharmacologic management indicated

Patient/Family Education
- Description of child's specific defect
- Strategies to promote normal development
- Information about nonpharmacologic management above

Outcomes and Follow-Up
- The child will participate in an early intervention program.
- The child will develop independence of self-care activities and mobility.
- The child will develop skills in other senses to compensate for lack of vision.
- The child will demonstrate socialization at home and school.
- The family will maintain a safe environment for the child.
- The family will orient the child to surroundings.
- The family will demonstrate strategies to promote optimal development.

CONJUNCTIVITIS

Description
Conjunctivitis is inflammation of the conjunctiva, the membrane lining the eyelid and covering the exposed surface of the sclera.

Etiology
The two common causes of bacterial conjunctivitis in children are *Streptococcus pneumoniae* and *Haemophilus influenzae*. Newborns may become infected during the birth process with *Chlamydia trachomatis* or *Neisseria gonorrhoeae*.

Incidence and Demographics
- About 15% of the population will have an episode of conjunctivitis at some time

Risk Factors
- Exposure to causative organism

Prevention and Screening
- No prevention or screening indicated

Assessment
- History of maternal infection

Physical Exam
- Crusty, purulent drainage
- Redness of the conjunctiva
- Swollen eyelid
- Burning sensation
- Itching
- Tearing

Diagnostic Studies
- Diagnosis based on symptoms
- Culture if no improvement

Management

Invasive
- No invasive management indicated

Nonpharmacologic
- Warm, moist compresses to loosen crusty drainage
- Cold compresses to decrease swelling
- Avoid eye makeup during infection
- Frequent handwashing

Pharmacologic
- *S. pneumoniae* and *H. influenzae*: Ophthalmic treatment
  - Erythromycin
  - Bacitracin/polymyxin B
  - Polymyxin B/TMP
- *C. trachomatis*
  - Erythromycin orally
- *N. gonorrhoeae*
  - Ceftriaxone (Rocephin) IM or IV
  - Cefotaxime (Claforan) IM or IV

Patient/Family Education
- Prevention of spread of infection
- Medication administration

Outcomes and Follow-Up
- The child will show decrease in redness, swelling, and drainage.
- The child and family will verbalize understanding of strategies to prevent spread of infection.
- The family will demonstrate medication administration.

OTITIS MEDIA AND OTITIS EXTERNA

Description
Acute otitis media (AOM) is a viral or bacterial infection of the middle ear. Otitis media with effusion (OME) is fluid in the middle ear without acute infection. Chronic suppurative otitis media is persistent infection resulting in perforation of the tympanic membrane. Otitis externa (OE), commonly called swimmer's ear, is bacterial infection of the outer ear.

Etiology
Obstruction of the Eustachian tube allows fluid to accumulate in the middle ear. The fluid may be contaminated from the nasopharynx, resulting in acute otitis media. If the fluid does not drain, an otitis media with effusion results. The effusion may last for weeks or months after the infection has resolved. Otitis media is often caused by *Streptococcus pneumoniae*, *Haemophilus influenzae*, and *Moraxella catarrhalis*. Most cases of chronic suppurative otitis media are due to penicillin-resistant *S. pneumoniae*.

The outer ear canal is ordinarily protected from infection by cerumen, but when the canal is altered by water, humidity, insufficient cerumen, or use of foreign object to clean canal, bacteria invade. Common causative organisms of otitis externa are *Pseudomonas*, *Enterobacteriaceae*, and *Proteus*.

Incidence and Demographics

Each year in the United States, 13.6 million pediatric office visits are for acute otitis media, and there are approximately 2.2 million cases of otitis media with effusion. The incidence of otitis media peaks in children between 6 and 24 months of age. It is more prevalent in Native Americans, Alaskans, and Canadian Inuit children. Otitis externa affects about 4 in 1,000 people annually. It peaks in children between 7 and 10 years of age.

Children are more prone to develop otitis media than adults for several reasons. The child's Eustachian tube is shorter, wider, lies more horizontal, and consists of underdeveloped cartilage. Children have larger adenoids that prevent drainage, immature humoral defense mechanisms leading to increased infection risk, and spend more time lying down which allows fluid to pool at the back of the throat with easy access to the Eustachian tube.

Risk Factors

Acute Otitis Media
- Bottlefeeding instead of breastfeeding
- Feeding in flat position rather than with head elevated
- Frequent contact with multiple children
- Exposure to tobacco smoke and air pollution
- Frequent pacifier use
- Previous episode of AOM
- Allergic rhinitis
- Cleft palate
- Down syndrome

Otitis Externa
- High humidity and warm temperatures
- Swimming
- Trauma to the ear canal
- Hearing aid use

Prevention and Screening
- No screening is indicated, but some prevention is possible.

Acute Otitis Media
- Breastfeeding
- Decrease use of pacifier in infants older than 6 months
- Avoid propping bottle
- Avoid exposure to tobacco smoke and pollution
- Avoid forceful nose blowing

Otitis externa
- Avoid using cotton swabs to clean ear canal
- Use hair dryer on lowest setting to dry canal after swimming or bathing
- Prophylaxis with acidifying or alcohol ear drops before swimming

Assessment
History
ACUTE OTITIS MEDIA WITH/WITHOUT EFFUSION
Upper-respiratory infection

OTITIS EXTERNA
Water in ear

Physical Exam
ACUTE OTITIS MEDIA
- Pain evidenced by ear pulling, head rolling, irritability in infants
- Immediate relief of pain if tympanic membrane ruptures
- Fever, rhinitis
- Decreased appetite, vomiting, diarrhea
- Postauricular and cervical lymph gland enlargement
- Tympanic membrane appears red, bulging, with no visible landmarks or light reflex

OTITIS MEDIA WITH EFFUSION
- Intermittent ear discomfort
- Feeling of fullness, popping, fluid motion
- Conductive hearing loss
- Tympanic membrane appears dull gray, slightly injected, with obscured landmarks and visible fluid level

CHRONIC SUPPURATIVE OTITIS MEDIA
- Signs of effusion

OTITIS EXTERNA
- Pruritus
- Pain
- Erythema
- Grayish, greenish, cheesy discharge
- Swelling with conductive hearing loss

Diagnostic Studies
- Tympanometry
- Tympanocentesis with aspiration and culture of middle ear fluid after multiple antibiotic failures

Management
Invasive
- Myringotomy with pressure-equalizing tube insertion

Nonpharmacologic
- Acute otitis media
- Application of heat or cold

Otitis Externa
- Clean canal of debris with curette
- Clean drainage from outer canal and skin around ear
- Apply petroleum jelly to skin around ear to prevent excoriation from drainage
- Gauze wick to get medication inside canal if canal is very edematous

Pharmacologic

OTITIS MEDIA
- Treatment for ear pain before initiation of antibiotic treatment
- Acetaminophen (Tylenol) or ibuprofen (Motrin)
- Analgesic ear drops such as antipyrine/benzocaine (Auralgan)
- Start antibiotics if symptoms persist
- Immediate antibiotic treatment for fever over 102.2° F (39° C), or for infant younger than 6 months of age
- First line: Amoxicillin (Amoxil, Trimox)
- Alternatives: Cefuroxime (Ceftin), cefdinir (Omnicef), cefprozil (Cefzil), azithromycin (Zithromax)
- Persistent OM: Amoxicillin/clavulanic acid (Augmentin), cefuroxime (Ceftin), ceftriaxone (Rocephin)

OTITIS EXTERNA
- Polymycin B/neomycin/hydrocortisone (Cortisporin otic drops)
- Ofloxacin (Floxin otic drops)
- Analgesics for pain

Patient/Family Education
- Diagnosis and treatment plan
- Medication administration
- Strategies for nonpharmacologic management
- Strategies for prevention
- Strategies for dealing with temporary conductive hearing loss
- Keeping water out of ears of children who have pressure-equalizing tubes

Outcomes and Follow-Up
- The child will experience effective pain management.
- The child will recover without complications.
  - Persistent hearing loss
  - Perforation of tympanic membrane
  - Acute mastoiditis
  - Delayed language development
- The family will verbalize understanding of diagnosis and treatment plan.
- The family will demonstrate medication administration, nonpharmacologic management, and strategies for dealing with hearing loss.
- The family will verbalize strategies for prevention.

RETINOBLASTOMA

Description
Retinoblastoma is a primary intraocular cancer.

Etiology
The disease begins with gene mutation. If untreated, retinoblastoma grows, causing retinal detachment and necrosis. Invasion continues into the orbit, the optic nerve, and then into the central nervous system. Sites of metastasis are lungs, bone, and brain.

Incidence and Demographics
The incidence of retinoblastoma is 1 in 20,000. It is usually diagnosed in children between 1 and 2 years of age, and onset after 5 years of age is rare.

Risk Factors
Family history

Prevention and Screening
There is no prevention, but screening for red reflex should be done at every well-child visit.

Assessment
History
- Family history
- Family often first to notice whitish glow

Physical Exam
- Leukokoria, white reflex instead of normal red reflex
- Strabismus
- Red eye
- Tearing
- Corneal clouding
- Discoloration of iris
- Blood in anterior chamber
- Glaucoma

Diagnostic Studies
- Indirect ophthalmoscopy to determine size and location of tumor
- Ultrasound
- CT scan
- MRI with contrast
- Lumbar puncture and bone scan in advanced disease

Management
Invasive
- Laser thermotherapy to destroy tumor with high temperature
- Cryotherapy to destroy tumor with extremely cold temperature
- Enucleation for advanced disease

Nonpharmacologic
- Radioactive plaques: High-dose radiation therapy
- External beam radiotherapy

Pharmacologic
- Chemotherapy to reduce tumor size before local therapy
- Vincristine (Oncovin)
- Cyclophosphamide (Cytoxan)
- Doxorubicin (Adriamycin)
- Cisplatin (Platinol)
- Carboplatin (CBDCA)
- Etoposide (VP-16, VePesid)

Patient/Family Education
- Diagnosis and treatment plan
- Side effects of chemotherapy
- Care of prosthetic eye

Outcomes and Follow-Up
- The child will recover without metastasis.
- The family will verbalize understanding of diagnosis and treatment plan.
- The family will demonstrate care of prosthetic eye.

TRAUMA TO THE EYE

Description
Eye trauma involves injury to the orbit, eyeball, eyelids, conjunctiva, or lacrimal glands.

Etiology
Orbital fractures are often caused by all-terrain vehicle (ATV) crashes, paintball injuries, and fireworks. Children most commonly sustain trapdoor, hinged orbital fractures. Penetrating injuries may be due to sharp objects such as scissors or knives, propulsive objects such as firecrackers or guns, or blunt objects such as small paintballs. Nonpenetrating trauma may be caused by foreign objects, chemical or thermal burns, or large balls. Trauma to the eye can lead to hyphema, an accumulation of blood in the anterior chamber, accompanied by increased intraocular pressure. After a few days, a secondary hemorrhage may occur with further increase in pressure and poorer chance of vision recovery. This secondary injury can cause glaucoma, vitreous hemorrhage, retinal detachment, choroidal rupture, sclera rupture, or otic atrophy. Another common result of trauma is corneal abrasion from contact lenses, foreign bodies, or chemicals. Corneal abrasion may lead to ulceration and erosion of the cornea with visual impairment.

Incidence and Demographics
- There are about 2.4 million eye injuries in the United States each year.
- Children under the age of 15 years account for one-third of eye trauma hospitalizations and 43% of all sports-related eye injuries.
- The most common injury is orbital fracture, accounting for about 39% of major eye trauma.
- 33% of children under the age of 6 years with hyphema develop secondary hemorrhage.

- The risk of secondary hemorrhage decreases with age and occurs more frequently in African Americans.
- Approximately 75% will recover visual acuity after hyphema treatment.
- 14% of individuals with hyphema will have poor visual results.
- Corneal abrasion is the most common eye injury and is most prevalent in those who wear contact lenses.

Risk Factors
- Lack of protective eyewear
- Participating in activity inappropriate for developmental age
- Sickle cell disease increases risk of increased intraocular pressure

Prevention and Screening
- Protective eyewear
- Adult supervision of dangerous activity

Assessment
- History of trauma
  ### Physical Exam
  ORBITAL FRACTURE
  - Intraorbital pain on eye movement
  - Diplopia, double vision, or blurred vision
  - Swelling
  - Nausea and vomiting

  HYPHEMA
  - Pain
  - Blurred vision
  - Photophobia
  - Tearing

  CORNEAL ABRASION
  - Pain or foreign body sensation
  - Tearing
  - Photophobia

  ### Diagnostic Studies
  - Visual acuity
  - Radiography or CT scan for suspected fracture
  - Slit lamp ophthalmic examination
  - Tonometry to measure intraocular pressure

Management
  ### Invasive
  - Suturing for lacerations
  - Surgical repair of fractures
  - Surgical evacuation of hyphema
  - Intraocular lens implantation for cataracts, a complication of trauma

Nonpharmacologic
HYPHEMA
- Eye patch and shield on affected eye
- Elevating head of bed 30° to 45° to promote settling of hyphema

CORNEAL ABRASION
- Ice compresses for 24–48 hours, then warm compresses
- Rest eyes

Pharmacologic
HYPHEMA
- Acetaminophen with or without codeine for pain
- Avoid aspirin and nonsteroidal anti-inflammatory drugs (NSAIDs)
- Topical aminocaproic acid (ACA, Amicar) to prevent secondary hemorrhage
- Topicals to decrease intraocular pressure
  - Brimonidine tartrate (Alphagan, Allergan)
  - Latanoprost (Xalatan, Pharmacia)
  - Timolol maleate (Timoptic-XE)

CORNEAL ABRASION
- Topical antibiotic to prevent infection
  - Ofloxacin (Ocuflox)
  - Polymyxin B/trimethoprim (Polytrim)
  - Ciprofloxacin (Cipro, Ciloxan)
  - Erythromycin (E-Mycin)
- Analgesics for pain
- Antibiotics to prevent infection
- Tetanus vaccine for penetrating injuries if not up to date
- Nonsteroidal anti-inflammatory eye drops
- Pain medication

Patient/Family Education
- Diagnosis and treatment plan
- Medication administration
- Nonpharmacologic management
- Prevention of future injury

Outcomes and Follow-Up
- The child will recover without permanent visual changes.
- The child and family will verbalize understanding of diagnosis and treatment plan.
- The child and family will verbalize understanding of nonpharmacologic management.
- The child and family will identify strategies to prevent future injury.
- The family will demonstrate medication administration.

REFERENCES

Abelson, M. B., Shapiro, A., & Lapsa, I. (2006). Meeting the challenge of conjunctivitis. *Review of Opthalmology, 51*, 78–81.

Abramson, D. H., Beaverson, K., Sangani, P., Vora, R. A., Lee, T. C., Hochberg, H. M., et al. (2003). Screening for retinoblastoma: Presenting signs as prognosticators of patient and ocular survival. *Pediatrics, 112*, 1248–1255.

Barclay, L., & Murata, P. (2008). *Nurse-administered anticipatory guidance may reduce ED visits for ear pain in toddlers.* Retrieved from http://www.medscape.com/viewarticle/569720

Batshaw, M. L., Pellegrino, L., & Roizen, N. J. (2007). *Children with disabilities.* Baltimore: Paul H. Brookes.

Burm, J. S. (2005). Internal fixation in trapdoor-type orbital blowout fracture. *Plastic and Reconstructive Surgery, 116*, 962–970.

Centers for Disease Control and Prevention. (2008). Healthy vision month—May 2008. *Morbidity and Mortality Weekly Report, 57*, 465.

Coco, A. S. (2007). Cost-effectiveness analysis of treatment options for acute otitis media. *Annals of Family Medicine, 5*(1), 29–38. Retrieved from http://www.medscape.com/viewarticle/553024

Hockenberry, M. J., & Wilson, D. (2007). *Wong's nursing care of infants and children.* St. Louis, MO: Mosby Elsevier.

Hoyt, K. S., & Haley, R. J. (2005). Innovations in advanced practice: Assessment and management of eye emergencies. *Topics in Emergency Medicine, 27*, 101–117.

Lazaridis, E., & Saunders, J. C. (2008). Can you hear me now? A genetic model of otitis media with effusion. *The Journal of Clinical Investigation, 118*, 471–474.

Melamud, A., Palekar, R., & Singh, A. (2006). Retinoblastoma. *American Family Physician, 73*, 1039–1044.

Osguthorpe, J. D., & Nielsen, D. R. (2006). Otitis externa: Review and clinical update. *American Family Physician, 74*, 1510–1516.

Patterson, B. L., & Anan, T. (2003). Facial trauma in a softball player. *Physician & Sportsmedicine, 31*(12), 26–29.

Ramakrishnan, K. K., Sparks, R. A., & Berryhill, W. E. (2007). Diagnosis and treatment of otitis media. *American Family Physician, 76*, 1650–1658.

Robertson, J., & Shilkofski, N. (Eds.). (2005). *The Harriet Lane handbook.* Philadelphia: Mosby.

Salvin, J. H. (2007). Systematic approach to pediatric ocular trauma. *Current Opinion in Ophthalmology, 18*, 366–372.

Sheppard, J. D. (2006). *Hyphema.* Retrieved from http://www.emedicine.com/oph/topic765.htm

Verma, A. (2008). *Corneal abrasion.* Retrieved from http://www.emedicine.com/oph/topic247.htm

9

Respiratory Disorders

Karen Corlett, MSN, RN-BC, CPNP-AC/PC, PNP-BC

DIFFERENCES IN PEDIATRIC ANATOMY AND PHYSIOLOGY

Infants are obligate nose breathers. Secretions or edema in the nasal passages significantly affect their comfort and ability to move air through the respiratory tree. Infants also have poorly developed intercostal muscles and pliable chest walls, resulting in inward motion (retractions) as they attempt to breathe more deeply. This maneuver can be counterproductive. Infant's airways are of a smaller caliber than their adult counterparts. Edema or the presence of secretions significantly impacts the size of the airway and increases the resistance to smooth air flow. One millimeter of tissue edema can decrease the effective airway size by 50% and increase resistance by a factor of 16 in small airways.

Anatomy
- Nose and mouth
- Nasopharynx
- Larynx
- Trachea
- Bronchi
- Bronchioles
- Alveoli
- Alveolar/capillary interface

Physiology

- Nose and mouth
  - Warmth
  - Humidity
  - Filtration by cilia
- Nasopharynx
  - Directs air to trachea, food to esophagus
- Larynx
  - Epiglottis protects airway
  - Vocal cords for vocalization and speech
- Trachea
  - Conductor of airflow
  - Warmth and humidification
- Bronchi
  - Conductors of airflow
- Bronchioles
  - Conductors of airflow
  - Muscular component to airway wall
    - Parasympathetic nervous system controls constriction and dilation of small airways
- Alveoli
  - Surfactant production
  - Surface area for gas exchange
- Alveolar/capillary interface
  - Diffusion of oxygen from alveolus to capillary
  - Diffusion of carbon dioxide from capillary to alveolus
  - Respiration accomplished here

Assessment

History

- Description of problem/symptoms
- Onset
- Duration
- Relieving or exacerbating events
- Current medications or treatments
- Past history

Physical Exam

- General appearance
- Chest wall
  - Shape
  - Retractions
    - Substernal, subcostal, intercostal, suprasternal
  - Pectus carinatum or excavatum
- Level of alertness
- Position of comfort
- Color
  - Central, peripheral

- Respiratory rate
  - Versus age-based expectations
- Respiratory effort
  - Use of accessory muscles
  - Retractions
  - Grunting
  - Flaring
- Respiratory patterns
  - Periodic breathing
    - · Can be normal in newborns
  - Apnea
    - · Pauses > 20 seconds
  - Prolonged inspiratory or expiratory phases
  - Depth of respirations
    - · Kussmaul respirations (rapid deep respirations without significant distress seen in diabetic ketoacidosis)
- Auscultation
  - Clarity and equality of breath sounds
  - Stridor
    - · Inspiratory phase
    - · Expiratory phase
    - · Biphasic stridor
  - Stertor
    - · Nasal congestion
  - Wheezes
    - · Obstruction to exhalation
    - · May disappear with severe obstruction due to lack of air movement across obstructed areas
  - Rales
    - · Small airway and alveolar component
  - Rhonchi
    - · Large airway noises from secretions or fluid

Diagnostics

- Arterial blood gas normals
  - pH   7.35–7.45
  - PaO2   80–100 mm Hg
  - PaCO2   35–45 mm Hg
  - HCO3   22–26 mEq/liter
  - Base Excess   -3 to +3
  - SaO_2 94%–100%
- Pulse oximetry
  - Noninvasive measurement of percentage of hemoglobin saturated with oxygen
- Culture of secretions/sputum
- Chest radiography
- Pulmonary function tests
- Laryngoscopy or bronchoscopy

BRONCIOLITIS/RESPIRATORY SYNCYTIAL VIRUS BRONCHIOLITIS

Description
Infection and inflammation of the small airways
- Cough, rhinorrhea
- Tachypnea
- Increased work of breathing
  - Retractions, flaring, or grunting
- Adventitious breath sounds
  - Crackles
  - Wheezes in some patients
- Hypoxemia in some
- Poor feeding in infants
- Young infants may present with apnea

Etiology
- Respiratory syncytial virus (RSV)
- Other viruses
  - Adenovirus
  - Influenza
  - Parainfluenzas
- Rare causes
  - *Mycoplasma*
  - *Chlamydia*
  - *Pneumocystis carinii*

Incidence and Demographics
- Most common cause of serious respiratory illness in infants
- Greatest occurrence in winter months
- 1%–3% of infants with bronchiolitis require hospitalization
  - Arterial oxygen desaturation best initial predictor of severe disease

Risk Factors
- Young infants with small airways and poor host defenses
- Ill contacts
- Prematurity or cardiopulmonary disease

Assessment
- Patency of (nasal) airway
  - Secretions
- Respiratory rate and effort
- Breath sounds
- Oxygen saturations
- Dehydration
  - Oral intake
  - Urine and stool output

- Moistness of mucous membranes
- Sunken fontanelle
- Skin turgor
- Peripheral pulses and perfusion
- Nasal washing to detect viral source
- Chest radiograph to exclude other pneumonic process
- Capillary or arterial blood gas if concern for respiratory failure

Management

Prevention

- Hand hygiene
- Segregation from sick contacts
- Prophylaxis for high-risk groups during winter months via passive immunization
  - Premature infants in first year of life
  - Infants with chronic cardiopulmonary compromise

Supportive Care

- Supplemental oxygen as indicated
- Intravenous hydration if indicated
- Fever control with acetaminophen

Bronchodilators Rarely Useful

- If ordered, assess before and after treatment for benefits

Parent Education

- Prevention
- Nasal airway clearance with bulb syringe
- Signs and symptoms of increasing respiratory compromise
- Signs and symptoms of dehydration
  - Acceptable intake and output
- Return for questions, deterioration, and for close follow-up

Outcomes and Follow-Up

- Close phone or office follow-up of nonhospitalized infants with bronchiolitis
- Most infants with short course and good recovery
- Bacterial co-infection possible
- Increased risk of hyperresponsive airways post-RSV infection

PNEUMONIA

Description

- Infection of the lung parenchyma
  - Characterized by infecting organism or mechanism
    - Bacterial, viral, aspiration
- Presenting symptoms are fever, cough, increased work of breathing, and/or shortness or breath
  - Range from mild dyspnea to toxic appearing child to respiratory failure

- Abnormal breath sounds
  - Decreased aeration, rales, and/or crackles
- Area of consolidation on chest radiograph
- Abdominal pain
  - Referred pain from pneumonia

Etiology and Demographics

- Newborns
  - Group B streptococcus, RSV
- Infants
  - Viruses
    - RSV, parainfluenza, influenza, adenovirus
  - Bacterial
    - *Bordatella pertussis, Streptococcus pneumoniae, Haemophilus influenzae, Mycobacterial tuberculosis*
    - *Chlamydia trachomatis* (vertical transmission)
- Preschoolers
  - Viruses
    - Parainfluenza and influenza virus, adenovirus, RSV
  - Bacterial
    - *Streptococcus pneumoniae, Mycobacterial tuberculosis*
    - *Mycoplasma pneumoniae*
- School age and older
  - Mycoplasma pneumoniae, Chlamydia pneumoniae
  - Bacterial
    - *Streptococcus pneumoniae, Bordetella pertussis, Mycobacterial tuberculosis*
- Immunocompromised patients
  - *Pneumocystis carinii*, fungal organisms, cryptococcal organisms

Risk Factors

- Vertical transmission (birth canal)
- Airway anomalies
  - Tracheoesophageal fistula
- Impaired airway clearance
  - Cystic fibrosis
  - Ciliary dysfunction
  - Ineffective cough
- Impaired barriers to infection
  - Tracheostomy tube
- Immunodeficiency or immunocompromise

Assessment

- Respiratory rate
- Work of breathing
- Breath sounds
- Fever
- Arterial oxygen saturation

- Associated illness
  - Bacteremia, meningitis, urinary tract infection
- Chest radiograph
- Secretions or nasal washing for viral or bacterial cause
- White blood cell count
- Ability to take oral food/fluids and maintain hydration

Management
- Antibiotics for suspected bacterial pneumonias
  - Based on age, chest x-ray, and symptoms
  - Oral for mildly ill children, parenteral antibiotics if more severely ill
  - Watch for resolution of fever
  - Consider evaluation for empyema if remains febrile on appropriate antibiotics
- Supportive care for suspected viral pneumonia
  - Rest, hydration, fever control
- Supplemental oxygen if hypoxia
- Intravenous hydration if unable to take oral fluids
- Evaluation of immune status if unusual organism isolated

Outcomes and Follow-Up
- Most respond to antimicrobial or supportive therapies well with no residual disease
- If fever persists, empyema as complication of bacterial pneumonia
  - May require surgical drainage
  - Lung function preserved in most

LARYNGOTRACHEOBRONCHITIS (CROUP)

Description
- Acute infection of the larynx and trachea
- Presenting symptoms
  - Preceded by mild upper-respiratory tract infection symptoms (cough, rhinorrhea, low-grade fever)
  - Parents describe harsh, croupy, brassy, barky, or seal-like cough
    · Noise worsens with agitation
    · May be relieved with cool air
  - Can progress to respiratory distress

Etiology
- Usually viral cause
  - Parainfluenzas most common
  - RSV, influenza, adenovirus, rubeola virus

Incidence, Demographics, and Risk Factors
- More common if previous episodes of croup
- Most common in fall and winter months
- Most frequent in infants and toddlers due to smaller airway size

Assessment

- History of upper-respiratory infection and description of cough
- Inspiratory stridor is classic finding
- Chest x-ray with "steeple sign" of narrowed airway
  - Not necessary for confirmation of disease
- Patency of airway
- Adequate ventilation and oxygenation
- Work of breathing, use of accessory muscles
- Do age and season fit suspected diagnosis?
  - Any concern for foreign body aspiration

Management

- Corticosteroids to decrease inflammation
  - Dexamethasone intramuscularly or enterally
- Inhaled racemic epinephrine to decrease airway edema/obstruction
  - Must observe posttreatment due to risk of recurrence after discharge
- Supplemental oxygen if arterial desaturation
- Inhaled helium/oxygen mixture to improve airflow delivery past obstruction and improve comfort
- Allow position of comfort
- Maintain hydration

Outcomes and Follow-Up

- Most episodes resolve over 2–4 days
- Steroids decrease duration of illness and hospitalizations
- Recurrence common
  - Educate family when to seek care

EPIGLOTTITIS

Description

- Life-threatening infection and inflammation of the epiglottis
- Sudden onset of high fever and systemic illness
- Toxic appearance, marked respiratory distress, and copious drooling
- Frightened, hyperalert, still child, hesitant to move head or neck
  - Classically sitting up with chin and neck thrust forward, mouth open and drooling

Etiology

- Classically, *Haemophilus influenzae* type B
  - Markedly decreased incidence since routine immunization
- Other causes
  - Nontypable *Haemophilus inflenzaes*, *Streptococcus pneumoniae* and *pyogenes*, staphylococcal organisms

Incidence and Demographics

- Classic age range: 2–5 years old
- Much less common since routine *Haemophilus influenzae* type B immunization began

Risk Factors
- Lack of immunization to *Haemophilus influenzae* type B

Prevention and Screening
- No prevention of screening indicated

Assessment
- Febrile, toxic-appearing, frightened child unable to swallow secretions with copious drooling and unusual posture
- Assessment should be stopped and care escalated as soon as diagnosis is suspected
- Any instrumentation of oral cavity or pharynx may cause life-threatening airway obstruction
- Airway x-ray may reveal classic "thumb sign" of swollen epiglottis
  - Risk of imaging high and benefit is low
- Elevated white blood cell count

Management
- To operating room with the most skilled pediatric anesthesiologist available to secure airway
  - Surgical airway team in place in case emergent tracheostomy required
- Pediatric intensive care management of artificial airway and respiratory failure
- Parenteral antibiotics to treat the likely bacterial infection

Outcomes and Follow-Up
- Excellent outcome if airway secured without period of hypoxemia
- Recurrence rare
- Return to routine pediatric care schedule
  - Consider assessment of immune status if *Haemophilus influenzae* type B infection confirmed and child has received immunizations
  - Immunization of the non- or under-immunized

FOREIGN BODY ASPIRATION

Description
- Aspiration of a foreign body into the respiratory tract
- Unwitnessed events present with sudden choking, coughing, and/or wheezing

Etiology
- Inhalation of food, toys, coins, or other small objects into the airway
- May cause partial or complete airway obstruction

Incidence and Demographics
- Highest incidence between 6 months and 4 years old

Risk Factors
- "Explorers" who mouth everything they find
- Small round foods
  - Nuts, grapes, hot dogs, carrots, hard candy
- Being active or mobile while eating/chewing

Prevention and Screening
- No prevention or screening indicated

Assessment
Complete Obstruction
- No air movement
- No noise with cough or attempted vocalizations
- Respiratory distress
- Progressive cyanosis
- Collapse
- Cardiopulmonary arrest

Partial Obstruction
- Cough
- Stridor
- Inspiratory and/or expiratory
- Dependent upon location of object
- Drooling
- Altered voice/cough quality
- Respiratory distress
- Unequal breath sounds if lodged in main stem bronchus

Management
- Activate the emergency medical system (EMS) and initiate basic and advanced life support as indicated
    - Blind finger sweeps not appropriate in infants or children since offending object may be advanced into the airway
- Alert, coughing victims should be allowed to attempt to clear their own airway while EMS is activated
    - Continuous assessment and monitoring for progression of obstruction
- Localization of foreign body
    - Chest radiograph may be helpful
- Direct bronchoscopy/laryngoscopy for foreign body removal
- Evaluation of injury to airway from object or instrumentation

Outcomes and Follow-Up
- Airway obstruction and resultant hypoxemia remains a significant cause of morbidity and mortality in pediatrics
- Follow-up of central nervous system or other end-organ injury if significant hypoxemia occurred with airway obstruction
- Caregiver evaluation and education about safe environment and safe eating/feeding practices

TONSILLITIS

Description
Inflammation and infection of the tonsils; may have associated infection in the throat (pharyngitis) as well.

Etiology
- Viral: Cause 90% of sore throats with fever
  - Peak incidence in summer and fall
  - Adenovirus, influenza, Epstein-Barr virus
- Bacterial: Cause 10% of sore throats with fever
  - Peak incidence in winter
  - Classic example and presentation of tonsillitis caused by Group A beta-hemolytic streptococcus
  - Other bacterial infections: Mycoplasma, *Haemophilus influenzae*

Incidence and Demographics
- Peak incidence between 5 and 15 years of age
- Rare in those under 2 years of age
- Most children will experience an episode of tonsillitis/pharyngitis at least once in childhood

Risk Factors
- Exposure to virus or bacteria causing tonsillitis
- Winter months
- School-age children have largest baseline tonsillar tissue so infection/inflammation may become most symptomatic

Prevention and Screening
- No prevention or screening indicated

Assessment
- Classic symptoms
  - Acute onset
  - High fever
  - Very sore throat, uncomfortable or difficult to swallow
  - Beefy red, inflamed tonsils
  - Pus on tonsils
  - Petechiae on palate
  - Foul-smelling breath
- Evaluate for alternative causes of illness
  - Associated systemic illness
  - Additional sites of infection
- Evaluate patency of airway
  - Ability to swallow
  - Voice quality
  - Respiratory distress
  - Altered level of consciousness

- Evaluation of causative organism
  - Rapid streptococcal screen
  - Confirm with culture, especially if initial screen negative

Management
- Group A beta-hemolytic streptococcus (GABHS) infection
  - Antibiotics
    · Almost universally susceptible to penicillins
    · Oral course, or single intramuscular depot injection
- Maintain hydration status
- Fever management

Outcomes and Follow-Up
- Excellent eradication of infection if full antibiotic course adhered to
- Education regarding the importance of taking the full course of antibiotics in a timely fashion
- Infectious complications
  - Peritonsillar abscess
  - Retropharyngeal abscess
- Post-GABHS infection complications
  - Postinfectious glomerulonephritis
  - Rheumatic fever

RESPIRATORY DISTRESS AND FAILURE

Description and Etiologies
- Spectrum of compromise to failure of gas exchange
- Inability to maintain adequate airway
  - Anatomic obstruction
  - Croup, epiglottitis, congenital malformation, airway trauma
  - Inadequate muscle control
  - Anesthesia, sedation, brain injury
- Inability to ventilate
  - Carbon dioxide diffuses easily at the alveolar level, so carbon dioxide levels may be normal even with significant parenchymal disease
  - Inadequate delivery of air to alveoli
  - Airway compromise
  - Air trapping
  - Asthma
- Inability to oxygenate
  - Alveolar disease
  - Pneumonia
  - Surfactant deficiencies
  - Pulmonary edema

- Failure to breathe
  - Apnea
  - CNS injury
  - Anesthesia, sedatives, neuromuscular blockers

Incidence and Demographics
- Dependent upon disease process

Risk Factors
- Young age
  - Smaller airways, fewer alveoli
- Preexisting cardiac or respiratory disease
  - Less reserve

Prevention and Screening
- No prevention or screening indicated.

Assessment
Physical Exam
- Respiratory rate
- Depth of respirations
- Respiratory effort
  - Use of accessory muscles
  - Retractions
  - Flaring
  - Grunting
- Breath sounds
  - Clarity and equality
  - Stridor
  - Wheezes
  - Rales
- Symmetry of chest expansion
- Palpation
  - Fremitus
    · Vibrations felt when palms on chest
    · Best if crying infant, or ask child to say "99"
    · Decreased fremitus/vibrations may indicate airway obstruction or fluid accumulation

Pulse Oximetry
- Measures adequacy of oxygenation

Blood Gas Analysis
- Respiratory acidosis
  - pH < 7.35, pCO_2 > 45—from inadequate ventilation
- Respiratory alkalosis
  - pH > 7.45, pCO_2 < 35—from hyperventilation

- Hypoxia
  - SpO_2 < 94% on room air
  - PaO_2 < 60–80mm Hg in infants; < 80–100mm Hg in children and adults

Management
- Dependent upon problem and disease process as described in this chapter
- Close observation for progression of respiratory distress
- Supplemental oxygen
- Noninvasive positive pressure ventilation
- Endotracheal intubation and mechanical ventilation

Outcomes and Follow-Up
- Dependent upon age, disease process, coexisting conditions
- Possibility of long-term sequelae to airways, lungs, or other organs

BRONCHOPULMONARY DYSPLASIA

Description
Chronic lung disease associated most often with prematurity

Etiology
- Premature birth
- Surfactant deficiency
- Lung injury
  - Meconium aspiration, infection, positive pressure ventilation

Incidence, Demographics, and Risk Factors
- Less common since advent of exogenous surfactant therapy for premature infants
- The more premature the birth, the higher the risk to the infant

Prevention and Screening
- Prevention
  - Prevention of premature birth
  - Corticosteroid therapy to mother prior to premature delivery
  - Exogenous surfactant administration to infant
  - Limitation of high pressures and volumes with mechanical ventilation

Assessment
- At 36 weeks postconceptual age, infant has all of the following:
  - Abnormal chest x-ray
  - Supplemental oxygen requirement
  - Abnormal respiratory exam (tachypnea, retractions, wheezes, rales, rhonchi, etc.)

Management
- Supplemental oxygen to maintain normal saturations
- Nasal continuous positive airway pressure (CPAP) or intubation and mechanical ventilation
- Diuretics
- Inhaled steroids, inhaled bronchodilators

Outcomes and Follow-Up
- Decreased mortality and morbidity from prematurity and chronic lung disease
- Increased risk of reactive airway disease and asthma if bronchopulmonary dysplasia
- Increased rate of hospitalizations in first 2 years of life
- Decreased somatic growth and development
- RSV prophylaxis if ordered
- Education for family
  - Signs and symptoms of respiratory distress
  - Home oxygen therapy and monitoring if necessary
  - Hand hygiene and infection control practices
  - When to seek care for exacerbations

CYSTIC FIBROSIS

Description
- Autosomal recessive genetic disorder
- Abnormal function of exocrine glands
  - Thick, tenacious airway secretions causing infections
  - Pancreatic insufficiency
    - Digestive enzymes
    - Insulin-dependent diabetes
    - Pancreatitis
- Abnormal sodium and chloride regulation
- Nasal polyps, frequent sinusitis, rectal prolapse all common

Etiology
- Autosomal recessive disorder

Incidence and Demographics
- Approximately 1/3,500 live births
- Most predominant in Whites of European ancestry

Risk Factors
- Genetic inheritance

Prevention and Screening
- No prevention or screening indicated

Assessment

Common Presentations/Concerning Symptoms

- Meconium ileus
- Failure to thrive
  - Bulky stools
- Frequent respiratory infections or pneumonias
  - Cough, productive cough
- Salty taste to skin
- Nasal polyps
- Recurrent sinusitis
- Hyperglycemia or diabetes
- Infertility

Diagnosis

- Sweat testing
  - Increased chloride content in collected sweat
- DNA testing
  - Serum testing for genetic mutations
  - Rare mutations may not be detected on routine screening
- Sibling screening if results positive

Management

- Multidisciplinary care team
- Respiratory
  - Thin and clear airway secretions
    - Hydration
    - Aerosolized medications
      · DNAse
      · Bronchodilators
    - Percussive therapies and postural drainage
    - Prevention and prompt clearance of lung infections
    - Lung tissue damaged further with each infection
    - Clear airways
    - Antibiotics as indicated—oral, intravenous, or aerosolized
      · Prophylactic antibiotics if ordered
    - Hand hygiene and infection-control measures
    - Appropriate infection-control measures if resistant organisms
  - Lung transplantation may be an option for progressive respiratory failure
- Dietary
  - Increased caloric intake
  - Pancreatic enzyme replacements
    - With each meal and snack to permit absorption of food
  - Vitamin supplements
    - Fat-soluble vitamins A, D, E, and K daily

- Pancreatic insufficiency
  - Glucose monitoring
    - Management of diabetes (see endocrine section)
- Rectal prolapse
  - Most common in infants
    - Due to frequent coughing, constipation
  - Manually reduce prolapsed tissue
  - Decrease fat and fiber in diet; administer stool softeners

Outcomes and Follow-Up
- Morbidities as above
- Life-shortening chronic disease
  - Lung damage resulting in progressive respiratory failure and death
  - Median life span now > 35 years
- Routine and impeccable pediatric and specialty care
  - Transition to adult providers at or before 21 years of age

TUBERCULOSIS

Description
Symptomatic infection with *Mycobacterium tuberculosis* complex

Etiology
Infection with one of the *Mycobacterium tuberculosis* complex bacteria
- Acid-fast, slow-growing bacilli

Incidence and Demographics
- 95% of tuberculosis occurs in developing countries
- More common in the immunocompromised
- Significant public health concern
  - Increasing multidrug resistance

Risk Factors
- Exposure to high-risk adults as below
- Those born in high-prevalence countries
- Homeless persons
- IV drug users
- Residents of nursing homes, shelters, and correctional institutions
- Healthcare workers caring for high-risk populations
- Immunocompromised persons

Prevention and Screening
- No prevention or screening indicated

Assessment
- Many infected children are asymptomatic
- Classic presentation/concerning symptoms
    - Fever
    - Cough
    - Weight loss or failure to thrive, anorexia, fatigue
    - Night sweats
- Tuberculin skin test
    - Induration is positive result (not just erythema)
    - Also will appear positive if received previous bacillus Calmette-Guerin immunization
- Highest risk of illness is first 1–2 years after infection
    - Infection can remain latent without signs and symptoms
    - Immunocompromise increases risk of disease
- Chest radiograph
    - To evaluate for pulmonary involvement
- Gastric lavage for culture 3 mornings in a row on empty stomach
    - Yield of positive culture remains low in children

Management
- Isoniazid plus rifampin for 6 months and pyrazinamide for 2 months is recommended regimen for children
- Observed medication administration recommended
    - Inconsistent antimicrobial therapy increases risks of resistant organisms
- Testing of contacts
- Prevention of spread
- Consider testing for HIV

Outcomes and Follow-Up
- Latent disease can become activated
- Severe pulmonary infections
    - Pleural effusions
    - Destruction of lung tissue
    - Spread into chest
- Spread outside of respiratory system
    - Bones and joints
    - Lymph system
    - Central nervous system
- Mandatory reporting to public health officials
- Meticulous medication administration
    - Education about rifampin
        - Orange appearance to body secretions
            - Stool, urine, tears, sweat
            - Will permanently stain contact lenses
- Monitoring for side effects of long-term medications

ASTHMA

Description
- Chronic inflammatory disorder of the airways
  - Inflammation of the airways
  - Airway hyperresponsiveness
  - Airflow obstruction

Etiology
- Genetic predisposition
- Allergic response
- Respiratory infections
  - Causation and trigger for worsening symptoms

Incidence and Demographics
- More common in Blacks than Whites
- ~12% of children have been diagnosed with asthma at some time in their lives
  - Incidence in United States continues to increase

Risk Factors
- Previous RSV infection
- Allergies and eczema
- Family history of asthma
- Smoke exposure

Prevention and Screening
- No prevention or screening indicated.

Assessment
History
- Cough, wheezing, chest tightness
- Worsening of above if exposed to triggers
- Smoke, animal dander, viral infections, dust, mold, pollens, change in weather

Physical Exam
- Expiratory wheezing
- Prolonged or forced expiratory phase
- Shortness of breath
- Respiratory distress

Atopic Symptoms
- Allergic "shiners" under eyes
- Eczema
- Rhinorrhea

Pulmonary Function Tests
- Forced expiratory volume in 1 second
- Compared to best predicted value
- Reversible airflow obstruction

Asthma Classification by
- Severity of disease
- Control of symptoms
- Responsiveness to therapy

Management
- Education on the disease, treatment, and triggers
  - Written asthma care plan
  - Indications to "step up" or "step down" therapies
    - As delineated on asthma care plan
- Routine monitoring of pulmonary function
- Identification and avoidance of triggers
- Long-term controller medications
  - Inhaled corticosteroids
    - First-line long-term controller medication
      - Rinse mouth after use to avoid thrush
    - Oral or parenteral steroids reserved for acute exacerbations
  - Inhaled long-acting beta agonists
    - Long-acting bronchodilator
    - Controller medication, not to be used for symptomatic relief
  - Mast cell stabilizers (cromolyn sodium)
  - Leukotriene inhibitors (monteleukast)
  - Immunomodulators (anti-IgE medications)
  - Methylxanthines (theophylline)
- Quick-relief medications
  - Inhaled short-acting beta agonists (albuterol)
  - Anticholinergics (ipatropium bromide)
- Inhaled drug delivery
  - Spacer/holding chamber
    - For use with metered dose inhalers
    - Increases percentage of dose delivered to lung
  - Nebulizer
    - If too young or unable to cooperate with spacer, or during acute exacerbations
    - Face mask for infants and young children
    - Mouthpiece for older children

Outcomes and Follow-Up
- Permanent airway remodeling can occur
  - Especially if poor control
- Periods of exacerbations and remissions
- Mortality from asthma on rise
- Parent/patient/provider partnership for control of asthma

SUDDEN INFANT DEATH SYNDROME (SIDS)

Description
- Sudden death of infant younger than 1 year of age without explanation
- Requires autopsy and investigation of death scene

Etiology
- Cause unclear, many associations under investigation
- Incomplete autopsy or death scene investigation may miss true causation of the sudden death

Incidence and Demographics
- Leading cause of death for infants 1–12 months of age
- Third leading cause of infant mortality in United States
- Marked decrease in overall incidence since "back to sleep" campaign initiated in 1990s

Risk Factors
- Prone or side sleeping
- Soft bedding or sleep surfaces
- Loose bedding
- Overheating
- Smoke exposure
- Bed-sharing
- Preterm and low birth weight

Prevention and Screening
- Prevention
  - Education on risk factors

Assessment
- The nurse is typically involved in the futile resuscitative efforts
- Awareness of the possibility of a SIDS diagnosis
  - Age
  - No other explanation for death
- Evaluation of reported story
  - Mandatory reporting if suspicion of abuse or neglect

Management
Support for Grieving Family
- Education and support for grieving siblings
- Assist family in informing siblings and extended family
- Allow family to be with, bathe, say goodbye to deceased infant
  - Assist in mementos
    - Footprints, handprints, lock of hair

Education on the Mechanism of SIDS
- No known cause
- Family did not cause death
- Local support groups may provide parent–counselors who have been through the experience of losing an infant to SIDS

Death Care
- Mandatory autopsy for sudden unexplained death
  - Medical examiner notification
- Notify organ/tissue retrieval organizations as per facility's policy
- Necessary paperwork
  - Funeral home name
- Prepare body for morgue per facility policy

Outcome and Follow-Up
Stages of Grief for Parents and Family
- Different members of family may grieve in different ways
- May be in different phases of grief at different times

Community Support
- Infant loss groups
- SIDS support groups
- Social, religious, and family supports
- Marriage counseling
  - Many marriages do not survive the loss of a child

REFERENCES

American Academy of Allergy, Asthma and Immunology. (2007). *Pediatric asthma guidelines.* Retrieved from http://www.aaaai.org/members/resources/practice_guidelines/pediatric_asthma.asp

Centers for Disease Control and Prevention & American Thoracic Society. (1999). *Diagnostic standards and classification of tuberculosis in adults and children.* Retrieved from http://www.cdc.gov/tb/pubs/PDF/1376.pdf

Centers for Disease Control and Prevention & Infectious Diseases Society of America. (2003). *Treatment of tuberculosis.* Retrieved from http://www.cdc.gov/mmwr/preview/mmwrhtml/rr5211a1.htm

Kliegman, R. M., Behrman, R. E., Jenson, H. B., Stanton, B. F. (Eds.). (2007). *Nelson's textbook of pediatrics* (18th ed.). Philadelphia: Saunders Elsevier.

National Health Center for Chronic Disease Prevention and Health Promotion, Division of Reproductive Health. (2009). *Sudden infant death syndrome and sudden unexpected infant death.* Retrieved from http://www.cdc.gov/SIDS/index.htm

Potts, N. L., & Mandleco, B. L. (Eds.). (2007). *Pediatric nursing: Caring for children and their families* (2nd ed.). Clifton Park, NY: Tomson.

Ralston, M., Hazinski, M. F., Zaritsky, A. L., Schexnayder, S. M., & Kleinman, M. E. (Eds.). (2007). *Pediatric advanced life support provider manual.* Dallas: American Heart Association.

Shah, I. (2006). *Pneumonias in children.* Retrieved from http://www.pediatriconcall.com/FORDOCTOR/DiseasesandCondition/Faqs/Pneumonia.asp

10

Cardiovascular Disorders

Karen Corlett, MSN, RN-BC, CPNP-AC/PC, PNP-BC

CONGESTIVE HEART FAILURE (CHF)

Description
Inadequate cardiac output to meet demands of the body

Etiology
- From structural heart disease
  - Extra blood flow to lungs steals blood flow from systemic circulation
  - Obstruction to systemic outflow
- From acquired heart disease
  - Coronary artery disease
  - Cardiomyopathy
  - Myocarditis
- Dysrhythmias
  - Inadequate pumping or inadequate filling

Incidence and Demographics
- Not well documented; see incidence and demographics for congenital heart disease

Risk Factors
- Structural heart disease
- Infections causing cardiomyopathy or myocarditis
- Ingestion of substances causing dysrhythmia
  - Previous dysrhythmia causing CHF

Assessment
For Causation
- Congenital heart disease
  - Electrocardiogram (ECG)
  - Cardiac ultrasonography
  - Rarely cardiac catheterization
  - Physical exam
- Cardiomyopathy or myocarditis
  - Cardiac ultrasonography for function
  - ECG for associated dysrhythmias
  - History
    · Of recent viral illness or ill contacts
    · Duration of symptoms
- ECG for presence of dysrhythmias

Physical Exam
- Cardiac
  - Tachycardia
  - Decreased peripheral pulses
  - Periorbital, peripheral, and/or dependent edema
  - Cool extremities
  - Delayed capillary refill
  - Hypotension a late sign
  - Cardiogenic shock in severe cases
- Pulmonary
  - Tachypnea
  - Increased work of breathing
    · Flaring, grunting, retracting
- Associated symptoms
  - Altered mental status if severe compromise
  - Decreased activity, increased sleep
  - Fussiness or irritability
  - Nausea, vomiting
    · Sweating with feeds in infants

Management
- Identification of problem as above

Medications
DIGOXIN
- For improved cardiac contractility and/or for some dysrhythmias
- Can load over 24 hours to speed accumulation of effective drug level
- Then dose orally twice daily for children, once daily for teens/adults
- Side effects
  - Bradycardia
  - Prolongation of PR interval
- Monitoring
  - Apical heart rate before dosing
  - Serum electrolytes: potassium, magnesium, calcium
  - Blood urea nitrogen (BUN), creatinine to evaluate for need of dosing
  - adjustments in renal insufficiency
  - For digoxin toxicity
    · Anorexia, nausea, vomiting, dizziness, bradycardia, heart block

DIURETICS
- To promote water loss and appropriate fluid balance
- Many can be dosed enterally or intravenously
- Loop diuretics
  - Affect sodium/potassium/chloride transport
  - Biggest effect in the ascending limp of the loop of Henle
  - Examples: furosemide, ethacrynic acid, bumetanide, torsemide
- Thiazide diuretics
  - Inhibit reabsorption of sodium and water in the distal convoluted tubules
  - Example: chlorothiazide
- Potassium-sparing diuretics
  - Inhibit action of aldosterone in the cortical collecting ducts
  - Example: chlorothiazide
- Monitoring
  - Serum electrolytes for losses with increased urine flow
  - Hyperkalemia a risk with potassium-sparing diuretics
  - Strict intake and output, daily weights
  - Hypotension or postural hypotension if large fluid shifts

AFTER LOAD REDUCERS
- Dilate peripheral vessels
  - Makes it easy for a poorly functioning heart to pump out systemically
  - Decreased peripheral vascular resistance favors more systemic outflow in patients with predominant left to right intracardiac shunting
  - Examples: enalapril, lisinopril

- Vastly different intravenous and oral dosage
- Monitoring
  - Hypotension with administration
  - Chronic cough
    · Renal function for dosing adjustments

NUTRITIONAL
- Hypercaloric formulas in infants
  - Consider tube feeding if unable to take adequate volumes
  - Careful monitoring for weight gain
  - Rarely need to restrict fluid or sodium intake
  - Education of parents re: potassium-rich foods if on diuretic therapy

INTENSIVE CARE MONITORING AND THERAPY IF POOR CARDIAC OUTPUT, SHOCK, OR RESPIRATORY FAILURE

SURGICAL CORRECTION OF STRUCTURAL HEART DEFECTS
- Cardiac transplantation if myopathy or myocarditis causes permanent heart muscle damage

FAMILY EDUCATION
- Signs and symptoms of worsening congestive heart failure symptoms as above
  - When to seek care
- Appropriate preparation of hypercaloric formulas
  - Tube feedings at home if ordered
- Medication administration
  - Medication safety—digoxin is quite toxic if ingested in inappropriate amounts
  - Signs and symptoms of digoxin toxicity as above

Outcomes and Follow-Up
- Goal is restoration of structure and function of heart muscle
- Normal cardiac output, organ, and peripheral perfusion
- Normal growth patterns
  - Height, weight, and development
- Close follow-up with pediatric cardiologist re: adjustment of medications
- Close follow-up with primary care provider re: growth and development
- Evaluation for any associated genetic abnormalities if congenital heart disease
  - Genetic counseling for families

CONGENITAL HEART DISEASE

Description
Structural abnormalities of the heart

Acyanotic Congenital Heart Disease
PATENT DUCTUS ARTERIOSUS (PDA)
- Persistence of ductus arteriosus
  - A normal prenatal structure connecting the aorta and the pulmonary artery
  - Allows for a "bypass" of the lung circulation in prenatal life when oxygenation is accomplished by the mother
  - Impetus for ductus to close is increase in oxygen tension
    · Also substances released from the lungs
    · Lack of exposure to maternal circulating prostaglandins
- More common in premature infants
  - And others with pulmonary issues
    · Causes left-to-right shunting
  - From high-pressured aorta to lower-pressure pulmonary artery
  - Pulmonary over-circulation
  - Steals from systemic circulation
  - Congestive heart failure
- Continuous murmur that radiates throughout chest

ATRIAL SEPTAL DEFECT (ASD)
- Hole or persistence of opening in the atrial septum
  - Connection between the right and left atria
  - Atria have low pressure, fairly equal between right and left side
- Some left-to-right shunting
  - Mild pulmonary over-circulation
  - Rarely causes significant congestive heart failure
- Murmur often absent or soft
  - Fixed split of S2 due to extra and constant flow across pulmonary valve

VENTRICULAR SEPTAL DEFECT (VSD)
- Hole in ventricular septum
  - Connection between the lower pumping chambers
  - After the newborn period the right ventricular pressure is only 20%–25% of left ventricular pressure
- Significant left-to-right shunting
  - Dependent upon size of hole
  - Can cause significant pulmonary over-circulation and steal from systemic circulation
  - Significant congestive heart failure in many
- Harsh, loud systolic murmur best at left lower sternal border

ATRIOVENTRICULAR CANAL DEFECT (AVC)

- Classified as an endocardial cushion defect
  - Failure of endocardial cushions to meet
    · Failure of migration of atrial and ventricular septum as well as abnormalities in formation of mitral and tricuspid valve tissue
    · More common in infants with Trisomy 21 (Down syndrome)
  - Range from tiny ASD with mitral valve abnormality and mild regurgitation to large ASD/VSD and essentially single valve separating atria from ventricles with significant regurgitation
- Predominant left-to-right shunting
  - Direction of shunting can be quite variable in large defects with multiple pathways for left-to-right shunting
  - Symptoms depend on size of holes and severity of valve involvement
  - Congestive heart failure common
- Harsh systolic murmur of VSD and/or systolic murmurs of tricuspid or mitral valve regurgitation

Cyanotic Congenital Heart Disease

TETRALOGY OF FALLOT

- Four "separate" defects arising from an abnormality in cardiac development
  - Ventricular septal defect
  - Pulmonary stenosis
    · At, below, or slightly above the pulmonary valve
  - Rightward malposition of the aorta
  - Right ventricular hypertrophy
    · Due to increased workload from pulmonary stenosis
- Cyanosis is predominant feature
  - Due to restriction of pulmonary blood flow
  - Deoxygenated blood in the right ventricle that can't get out across stenotic pulmonary valve crosses the VSD into the left ventricle and exits as deoxygenated blood into the systemic circulation via the aorta
  - Systolic ejection murmur from turbulence across stenotic pulmonary valve

TRANSPOSITION OF THE GREAT ARTERIES (TGA)

- Also known as "simple transposition"
  - The aorta arises from the right ventricle and the pulmonary artery arises from the left ventricle
  - Creates two "separate" rather than "in series" circulations
    · Deoxygenated blood travels from inferior and superior vena cava, to right atria, to right ventricle, to the aorta, to the lungs
    · Oxygenated blood returns from the lungs via the pulmonary veins to the left atria, to left ventricle and back to the pulmonary artery to the lungs
    · Potential connection points to mix the blue and red blood are the PDA and the persistence of the prenatally present foramen ovale connecting the right and left atria
- Mandatory cyanosis
  - Can have pulmonary over-circulation as well
- Murmur may be unimpressive
  - Only turbulent blood flow is across PDA and/or ASD

TRUNCUS ARTERIOSUS
- Single common "trunk" exits the heart
  - "Trunk" continues out and becomes aorta, gives rise to the pulmonary arteries
    · Classified by how the pulmonary arteries come off of main trunk
  - Implies ventricular septal defect as well
    · "Trunk" originates over the VSD
  - Valve to truncal vessel has components of aortic and pulmonary valves and can be malformed as well
- Causes pulmonary over-circulation and cyanosis
  - Deoxygenated blood from the right side of the heart and oxygenated blood from the left side mix completely together at the VSD and exit the truncal
    · This mixed blood then follows the path of least resistance
      - Some will go to the pulmonary artery connection back to the lungs
      - The remainder will continue out the aorta to give cardiac output to the body
    · As the pulmonary artery pressures of a newborn drop, more blood will travel to the lower-pressure pulmonary arteries
  - Congestive heart failure, cyanosis, and low cardiac output can coexist
- Murmur varies
  - Of stenosis or regurgitation across truncal valve
  - Right and left ventricles are fairly equal in pressure so not a lot of turbulent blood flow across the VSD

TRICUSPID ATRESIA
- Tricuspid valve never formed
  - No opening between right atria and right ventricle
  - Typically have small, underdeveloped hypoplastic right ventricle
  - May have VSD and/or pulmonary stenosis as well
  - Right ventricle will never be usable as a pump
    · This is a type of "single ventricle"
- Cyanosis
  - No blood flow into right ventricle so no blood flow through pulmonary valve into pulmonary artery and to lungs
- Murmur may not be impressive—mostly from PDA and ASD unless other anomalies

TOTAL ANOMALOUS PULMONARY VENOUS RETURN (TAPVR)
- The pulmonary veins end up in the wrong place
  - Pulmonary veins bring highly oxygenated blood back from the lungs
  - Should enter as four separate vessels into the back of the left atrium
  - In TAPVR the vessels typically come together behind the left atrium, then travel through an abnormal vessel to somewhere in the right heart
    · Categorized by the course and/or entrance point of the pulmonary veins back into the heart
  - Implies an ASD

- Pulmonary circulation and cyanosis of varying degrees
  - Recirculation of oxygenated blood back through the right side causes pulmonary over-circulation
  - Because no blood is coming back to the left atrium, there is a mandatory right-to-left shunt at the atrial level
    · Provides blood flow to the left ventricle for cardiac output
    · Deoxygenated blood from the right atrium enters into the systemic circulation
  - If there is narrowing or obstruction of the pulmonary veins on their course back to the heart, infants will present in cyanosis and shock
  - TAPVR may be an isolated condition, or may be just a portion of a complex congenital heart deformity
- Not an impressive murmur

Obstructive Lesions

PULMONARY STENOSIS
- Isolated stenosis of the pulmonary valve
- Limits pulmonary blood flow
- Increased pressure, work load, and thickness of right ventricle
- Rarely causes cyanosis
- Systolic ejection murmur from turbulent flow across pulmonary valve

AORTIC STENOSIS
- Isolated stenosis or narrowing of the aortic valve
- Can limit blood flow out to the body
- Increased pressure, work load, and thickness of the left ventricle
- Can cause poor cardiac output
- Systolic ejection murmur from turbulent flow across narrowed aortic valve

COARCTATION OF THE AORTA
- Narrowing of the aorta
- Typically just across from the left subclavian artery
- Newborns present in shock
- Older children present with some or no symptoms
  - Hypertension on routine blood pressure checks
    · High right arm pressures before obstruction, lower or normal blood pressure of left arm or legs
  - Leg cramps
- Increased pressure, work load, and thickness of left ventricle
- May have no murmur

HYPOPLASTIC LEFT HEART SYNDROME (HLHS)
- All left-sided structures are small or atretic
  - Mitral valve, left ventricle, aortic valve, and ascending aorta
  - Left side is unusable as a pump for systemic circulation
    · Ascending aorta is inadequate for systemic outflow

– Oxygenated blood returning to left atrium crosses from the left atrium to the right atrium, joins the deoxygenated blood returning from the body; this mixed blood enters the right ventricle and is pumped out the pulmonary valve into the pulmonary artery
  · The blood then:
    ▪ Can go through the PDA to the aorta to supply the body with blood flow
    ▪ Can continue out the right and left pulmonary artery and go to the lungs to become fully saturated and return to the left atrium
    ▪ Constant balance between the amount of pulmonary vs. systemic blood flow
  – Is a type of single ventricle
• Requires a connection between the right and left atrium so the blood returning from the lungs can cross to the right side
• Requires the ductus arteriosus to stay open to provide systemic blood flow
• Minimal to no murmur despite severity of disease

Etiology
• As yet, no clearly defined environmental and genetic factors
• Maternal infections during pregnancy
• Teratogenic drugs including alcohol

Incidence and Demographics
• 0.7/1,000 live births
• ~35,000 infants each year born in the United States with congenital heart disease
• Largest cause of infant death compared to all other birth defects

Risk Factors
• Intrauterine exposure to drugs, alcohol, or infections
• Previous child with congenital heart disease
• Parent with congenital heart disease
• Associated genetic syndromes
  – Down syndrome
  – Williams syndrome
  – Turner syndrome
  – Noonan syndrome
  – Trisomy 13 and 18

Prevention and Screening
• No prevention or screening indicated

Assessment
Cardiac Exam
• Heart rate vs. normal for age and condition
  – Higher if febrile, crying, active, or dehydrated
• Heart rhythm

- Presence of murmur
  - Grade or loudness (I through VI scale)
    - Grade I: Softer than heart tones
    - Grade II: Equal in intensity to heart tones
    - Grade III: Louder than heart tones
    - Grade IV: Louder than heart tones and there is a palpable thrill
    - Grade V: Grade IV criteria and heard with stethoscope partially off chest
    - Grade VI: Grade IV criteria and heard with stethoscope off chest
  - Location best heard
    - In relation to:
      - Sternum
      - Clavicle
      - Axillae
      - Intercostal spaces
  - Quality
    - Harsh, blowing, machinery, soft, click
  - Timing
    - During systole
    - During diastole
  - Additional sounds
    - S3 (Sounds like "Kentucky")
    - S4 (Sounds like "Tennessee")
    - Pericardial rub (From pericardial inflammation and/or fluid accumulation)
- Evaluation of peripheral perfusion
  - Central and peripheral pulses
  - Peripheral warmth
  - Central and peripheral color
  - Cyanosis or pallor
  - Capillary refill time
  - Sweating
- Evaluation of cardiopulmonary interactions
  - Hepatomegaly
  - Respiratory rate and effort
  - Pulmonary edema
- Presence of edema
  - Periorbital
  - Peripheral
  - Dependent
  - Pulmonary
  - Strict intake vs. output measurements
- Point of maximal impulse
- Jugular venous distention

Cyanosis
- Central and peripheral
- Noninvasive pulse oximetry
- Invasive arterial blood gas

Pulmonary Over-Circulation
- Respiratory exam
- Chest radiography

Impact on Other Systems

FATIGABILITY
- Sleeping and eating in infants
- Endurance in older children

GROWTH
- Decreased intake due to rapid fatigue
- Increased caloric requirements due to increased workload on heart

DEVELOPMENT
- Delayed developmental milestones due to fatigue
  - Of increased work of breathing
  - Of increased cardiac workload
  - Of poor caloric intake

OTHER ORGAN SYSTEMS
- Decreased perfusion from inadequate cardiac output can affect the functioning of any other organ system
  - CNS: Confusion, sleepiness, lethargy
  - Renal: Increased BUN/creatinine, decreased urinary output
  - Hepatic: Decreased hepatic function, increased laboratory parameters (liver enzymes and coagulation studies)
  - Gastrointestinal: Edematous, boggy intestinal walls with poor absorption

EVALUATION OF CONGENITAL HEART DEFECTS
- ECG and cardiac exam point to problem
- Cardiac echocardiography
  - Noninvasive test to look at structure and function of heart
  - Requires sedation or distraction for infants and young children to cooperate
- Cardiac catheterization
  - Typically via femoral artery and/or vein
  - Catheters advanced and contrast injected into bloodstream
    - Look at structure and function
    - Direct measurements of pressures and oxygen saturations within the heart
  - Typically receive sedation or anesthesia for procedure
- Cardiac magnetic resonance imaging (MRI)
  - Noninvasive study to look at cardiac structures
  - Infants and young or uncooperative children need sedation or anesthesia to accomplish study

Management

- Management of congestive heart failure as above
  - Optimize cardiac output
  - Optimize balance between pulmonary and systemic circulations
  - Optimize nutrition and growth
  - Avoid intercurrent infections
- Surgical repairs
  - Some defects now treated with cardiac catheterization
    - PDA closures
      - In all but neonates
      - Coils delivered by catheter and placed in PDA
    - ASD closure
      - Device placed by catheter in the ASD
      - Patient must be big enough for safe placement of large catheter to deliver device
    - Opening of stenotic pulmonary or aortic valves
      - Catheter passed across valve and balloon blown up to widen outflow
    - Postprocedure monitoring
      - Bleeding from catheter entry points
      - Extremity straight and still as ordered postprocedure
      - Perfusion distal to catheter entry points
      - Signs and symptoms of infection at catheter entry points
  - Most require cardiopulmonary bypass (CPB)
    - The heart can be stopped, opened, and worked on with maintenance of oxygenation and blood flow to the tissues
      - The heart itself does not receive blood flow
    - Avoids entry of air into the circulation when heart opened
    - Requires blood thinner to limit clotting in the bypass circuit
    - PDA and coarctation of aorta do not require cardiopulmonary bypass
    - CPB initiates a systemic inflammatory response (to the artificial tubing and machinery)
  - Most repairs via midline sternotomy incision
    - Chest tubes for drainage of thorax post-op
      - Maintenance of suction and/or water seal
      - Avoidance of leaks in system
      - Careful record of amount and consistency of drainage
    - Dressing changes as ordered
    - Early identification and treatment of local and deep infections
    - 4–6 weeks of limited activities to avoid injury/reinjury to healing sternum
    - May have temporary pacing wires in place
      - In case of dysrhythmia
    - Promote coughing, deep breathing, walking for pulmonary toilet once off mechanical ventilator
    - PDA and coarctation most often via lateral thoracotomy
  - Single-stage repairs
    - Full repair with one surgery

- Palliations with multistage repairs
  - Shunts or bands to augment or limit pulmonary blood flow
    - May not have "normal" oxygen saturations after palliations
  - Later full repair or
  - Continuation of staged repairs
  - Many complex congenital heart defects never can be fully repaired
    - Goal is to minimize workload on heart
    - Achieve near-normal systemic saturations
    - Create best repair that is surgically possible
  - Cardiac transplantation may be an option

Outcomes and Follow-Up
- Failure of medical management of CHF
  - Points to timing for surgical repair
- Surgical morbidity and mortality
  - Highly dependent on age of child, condition, congenital defect, associated anomalies
  - Reoperations required for some
    - Replacement of nongrowing tissues
    - Readdressing narrowed or regurgitant valves
    - Residual holes
- Postoperative infections
  - Rare but can be additional cause of morbidity and mortality
- Lifelong follow-up with cardiologist
  - Even if uncomplicated full repair
- Routine follow-up with primary care provider
- Bacterial endocarditis prophylaxis
  - For those with significant residual heart disease or implanted artificial material
  - Antibiotics immediately before and after procedures that create high risk of introducing bacteria into the blood stream

KAWASAKI DISEASE

Description
- An acute, systemic vasculitis in children
- Characterized by:
  - Fever
  - Rash
  - Conjunctivitis
  - Inflammation of the mucus membranes
  - Swollen lymph glands in the neck
  - Inflammation of arteries

Etiology
- Not well-understood
- Likely genetic predisposition + environmental trigger
  - May be postinfectious but mechanism not well delineated

Incidence and Demographics
- About 4,000 cases in the United States each year
- 80% of patients < 5 years of age
- Boys > girls

Risk Factors
- Asian ancestry at higher risk

Prevention and Screening
- No prevention or screening indicated

Assessment
- Classic symptoms:
  - High fever
  - Rash
  - Swollen hands and feet with peeling of palms and soles
  - Conjunctivitis: irritation and redness of sclera
  - Swollen lymph glands in the neck
  - Swollen, red, dry, cracked, and peeling lips
  - Red, coated, pitted, inflamed tongue ("strawberry" tongue)
- May have new murmur but rare
- Cardiac echocardiography to evaluate coronary arteries
  - Coronary aneurysms can develop
  - Typically develop over time, not often present at beginning of illness
- Evaluation for other cause of illness
  - Blood and urine cultures often sent

Management
- Identification of disease as above
  - Cardiology and infectious disease specialists often involved
- Education of family about disease process and treatments
- Intravenous immunoglobulin
  - Pretreatment with acetaminophen and/or diphenhydramine as ordered
  - Administer per hospital policy
  - Careful titration of rate of infusion as per hospital policy
    - Large volume to infuse, monitor intake vs. output, urine output, and cardio respiratory exams closely during infusion
- Aspirin
  - For anti-inflammatory effects
  - Education of family to not use aspirin for routine fever/pain management due to risk of Reye's syndrome
- Continued surveillance with echocardiogram for development of coronary artery aneurysms

Outcomes and Follow-Up
- Mortality < 1%
- Recurrence rare (< 2%)
- 15%–25% with coronary sequelae
  - Continued aspirin therapy if coronary artery aneurysms present
- Emphasize importance of lifelong specialty care follow-up

RHEUMATIC FEVER

Description
- Acute, inflammatory, autoimmune complication of Group A beta hemolytic streptococcal (GABHS) infection
- Characterized by joint pain, chorea, attack of the heart valves, skin nodules

Etiology
- Autoimmune response
- Post-GABHS infection—classically "strep throat"
  - Often untreated or incompletely treated GABHS infection

Incidence and Demographics
- 5- to 15-year-olds with highest incidence
  - Higher rates of GABHS infection
- No currently available statistics for rates of attack
- Much more common in developing countries

Risk Factors
- Untreated or undertreated GABHS infection
- Previous occurrence of rheumatic fever

Prevention and Screening
- No prevention or screening indicated

Assessment
- Typical physical findings
  - Red, cracked, dry, inflamed, peeling lips
  - Conjunctival injection
  - Strawberry tongue
  - Tender joints
    - May be unwilling to walk
    - Multiple joints involved
    - Affected joints can change daily
  - Swollen, inflamed hands and feet with peeling of soles and palms
  - Chorea: Random gyrating movements of body
    - Late symptom but on occasion is only symptom

- New murmur
  - Or acquired heart disease on cardiac echocardiography
- ECG changes
  - Prolonged PR interval most common abnormality
- Evidence of inflammation
  - Elevated erythrocyte sedimentation rate (ESR) or C-reactive protein (CRP)
- Evidence of recent streptococcal infection
  - Positive throat culture
    - Rapid test not enough
  - Rising antistreptolysin titer (ASO)
- Evaluation for other causes
  - Infections
  - Autoimmune diseases such as juvenile rheumatoid arthritis

Management
- Antibiotics to eradicate the streptococcal infection
- Aspirin as anti-inflammatory
  - Rapid improvement with initiation of aspirin
  - Antacids for stomach protection
- Bed rest until resolution of acute inflammation

Outcomes and Follow-Up
- Rheumatic heart disease and rheumatic fever caused > 3,200 deaths in 2004—all ages
- Activity limitations depend on degree of heart damage
  - Attack is usually to the valves
  - Mitral and aortic valves most susceptible
  - Risk of further valve disease with repeated attacks of rheumatic fever
- High incidence of recurrent attacks
  - Secondary prophylaxis
    - Continued therapy with penicillin
    - For at least 10 years since last attack *and* at least until 21 years of age
- In-depth education and discussion re: importance of penicillin regimen and risk of recurrent attack
  - Difficult to maintain daily drug therapy when child is well and feels fine
  - Daily oral medication or monthly depot injections
    - May try different forms at different ages and developmental stages
    - Advantage of thinking about therapy only once monthly vs. pain of injection
- Continued follow-up with pediatric cardiologist, then transition to adult cardiology care providers

REFERENCES

American Heart Association, Committee on Rheumatic Fever, Endocarditis, and Kawasaki Disease, Council on Cardiovascular Disease in the Young. (2004). Diagnosis, treatment, and long-term sequelae of Kawasaki disease. *Circulation, 110,* 2747–2771.

Hazinski, M. F. (Ed.). (1991). *Nursing care of the critically ill child.* Philadelphia: Mosby.

May, L. E. (2005). *Pediatric heart surgery: A ready reference for professionals.* Milwaukee, WI: Maxishare.

Park, M. K. (Ed.). (2008). *Pediatric cardiology for practitioners.* Philadelphia: Mosby Elsevier.

Potts, N. L., & Mandleco, B. L. (Eds.). (2007). *Pediatric nursing: Caring for children and their families* (2nd ed.). Clifton Park, NY: Tomson.

Takemoto, C. K., Hodding, J. H., & Kraus, D. M. (2007). *Pediatric dosage handbook* (14th ed.). Hudson, OH:: Lexi-Comp.

Zieve, D. & Fogel, M. A. (2007). *Congenital heart disease.* Retrieved from http://www.nlm.nih.gov/medlineplus/ency/article/001114.htm#Causes,%20incidence,%20and%20risk%20factors

Gastrointestinal Disorders

Clara J. Richardson, MSN, RN-BC

CLEFT LIP AND PALATE

Description
Cleft lip is defined as unilateral or bilateral separation of the upper lip that may extend into the upper jaw and the upper gum. Cleft palate is an opening in the roof of the mouth involving just the soft palate or both soft and hard palates.

Etiology
Orofacial clefts are due to lack of cellular growth and/or failure of fusion during the embryonic period. It is estimated that 3 to 14 genes contribute to cleft lip and palate. Lip formation occurs between the sixth and eighth weeks of gestation, while palate formation takes place between the seventh and twelfth weeks.

Incidence and Demographics
The incidence of cleft lip, with or without cleft palate, is 1 in 700 live births, and is more common in males. Cleft palate without cleft lip has an incidence of 1 in 2,500 live births and is more common in females.

Cleft lip and palate occurs more frequently in Northern Europeans, Asians, Native Americans, and Aboriginal Australians. Cleft lip alone occurs more frequently in Africans and those of African descent.

Recent research has shown that individuals with orofacial clefts have shorter life spans, increased risk of hospitalization for psychiatric diseases as adults, increased occurrence of breast and brain cancer among adult females, and increased occurrence of lung cancer among adult males.

Risk Factors
- Maternal use of corticosteroids during early pregnancy
- Maternal cigarette smoking during pregnancy
- Maternal folic acid deficiency during pregnancy
- Maternal use of phenytoin (Dilantin) or valproic acid (Depakote, Depakene) during pregnancy
- Maternal exposure to solvents such as carbon tetrachloride, tetrachloroethylene, trichloroethylene; triazine herbicide; pollutants such as chloroform, methyl mercury, and hazardous waste products during pregnancy

Prevention and Screening
Prevention is aimed at avoidance of risk factors during pregnancy, specifically smoking, corticosteroid use, and phenytoin use. Prepregnancy folic acid supplement is advised. Screening involves examination for physical signs in all newborns.

Assessment
History
- Familial history
- Prenatal history

Physical Exam
- Visualization of cleft lip
- Visualization or palpation of cleft palate
- Nasal regurgitation of feeding

Diagnostic Studies
- May be diagnosed in utero on ultrasound by 14–16 weeks gestation

Management
Invasive
- Cleft lip adhesion at 6 weeks
- Cleft lip repair at 3 months
- Cleft palate repair at 12 months
- May involve several revisions by plastic surgeon to improve physical appearance
- May need myringotomy tube placement due to frequent bouts of otitis media
- May require bone grafts to support teeth and palate revisions to correct hypernasal speech

Nonpharmacologic
- Orthodontist to realign teeth
- Audiologist to evaluate for hearing defects
- Speech pathologist to treat speech problems
- Mental health professional to support child and family coping
- Preoperative care
  - Variation of position for breastfeeding
  - Use of breast pump to initiate let-down
  - Special nipples, bottles, squeezable tubes
  - Practice with postoperative feeding methods and restraints

Postoperative Care
- Avoid prone position with cleft lip repair
- Possibly elbow restraints to prevent suture irritation
- Avoid objects in mouth such as pacifiers, straws, spoons after cleft palate repair
- Clean lip sutures with saline and rinse mouth after feedings
- Liquid or pureed foods after cleft palate repair

Pharmacologic
- Postoperative pain management
- Possibly postoperative sedation to keep infant calm and prevent strain on lip sutures from crying
- Antibiotic ointment on lip suture line

Patient/Family Education
- Feeding techniques
- Signs of dehydration and inadequate nutritional intake
- Postoperative care
- Pain management

Outcomes and Follow-Up
- The infant will show no signs of dehydration.
- The infant will exhibit adequate growth.
- The infant will attain normal developmental milestones.
- The infant is comfortable and rests quietly with effective pain management.
- The family will exhibit attachment behaviors.
- The family will verbalize understanding of defect and treatment plan.
- The family will demonstrate successful feeding strategies.
- The family will demonstrate postoperative care strategies.
- The family will return for regular follow-up with the craniofacial team.

TRACHEOESOPHAGEAL FISTULA (TEF) AND ESOPHAGEAL ATRESIA (EA)

Description
Tracheoesophageal fistula (TEF) is a congenital malformation consisting of a connection between the trachea and the esophagus. In a related congenital defect, esophageal atresia (EA), the esophagus ends in a blind pouch with no connection to the stomach. These may occur separately, but most often occur in combination.

Etiology
Respiratory and digestive tubes develop into distinct structures at approximately day 22 of gestation. When this development is disrupted, TEF and/or EA occur.

Incidence and Demographics
The incidence of these defects is 1 in 2,400–4,500 live births; 88.5% of cases involve both TEF and EA. Isolated EA accounts for 8% of cases and isolated TEF for another 4%. The remaining cases consist of rare structural combinations. Approximately 25% of these infants have other congenital anomalies in the cardiac, genitourinary, gastrointestinal, skeletal, and/or central nervous system.

Risk Factors
- Prematurity
- Low birth weight

Prevention and Screening
No specific prevention has been identified. Screening consists of identification of pertinent history and physical signs, preferably before first feeding. An attempt to pass a feeding tube will be unsuccessful and further diagnostic testing should begin.

Assessment
History
- Maternal history of polyhydramnios, excess amniotic fluid
- Prenatal ultrasound without visualization of stomach

Physical Exam
PREOPERATIVE FINDINGS
- Excessive mucus
- Coughing, choking, cyanosis on feeding
- Respiratory distress with rales

POSTOPERATIVE FINDINGS
- Signs of leak at suture line include respiratory distress or sepsis
- Signs of stricture include coughing, regurgitation, recurrent aspiration
- Signs of stricture after immediate postoperative period include failure to thrive, difficulty swallowing, dysphagia

Diagnostic Studies
- Radiography
- Contrast studies
- Bronchoscopy

Management
Invasive
- Surgical division of the TEF and anastomosis of the esophagus
- In cases when the ends of the esophagus are too short to connect, anastomosis is delayed until growth occurs
- Temporary cervical esophagostomy allows drainage of secretions and gastrostomy tube feedings provide nutrition until repair

Nonpharmacologic
- Preoperative care
  - Intermittent or continuous suction to clear secretion in pouch
  - Upright or prone position at 30 degrees
  - Thermoregulation
  - Skin care with esophagostomy
- Postoperative care
  - Premeasured and marked catheter for suctioning
  - Radiant warmer
  - Chest tube
  - Nasogastric tube
  - Parenteral nutrition
  - Progression to oral or gastrostomy feedings
- Treatment of stricture is esophageal dilation

Pharmacologic
- Preoperative antibiotics to treat or prevent aspiration pneumonia
- Postoperative pain management

Patient/Family Education
- Explanation of defect and treatment plan
- Home care including feeding technique, promotion of normal development
- Signs of complications
- Cardiopulmonary resuscitation and choking relief

Outcomes and Follow-Up
- The child will maintain a patent airway with effective respirations.
- The child will maintain effective thermoregulation.
- The child attains appropriate growth and developmental milestones.
- The child will not experience complications such as leak at anastomosis, esophageal stricture, dysphagia, gastroesophageal reflux disease, tracheomalacia, recurrent respiratory infection, recurrent TEF, or pulmonary function abnormalities.

- The family will verbalize understanding of defect and treatment plan.
- The family will demonstrate home care strategies.
- The family will identify signs of complications.
- The family will verbalize understanding of CPR and choking relief.

IMPERFORATE ANUS

Description
Imperforate anus is a congenital anorectal malformation with varying degrees of severity classified as low, intermediate, or high. The rectum may end in a blind pouch or it may have fistulas to the genitourinary system or to the perineum.

Etiology
This defect is due to abnormal fetal development during the sixth week of gestation when the rectum fails to assume its normal position.

Incidence and Demographics
Imperforate anus occurs in approximately 1 in 4,000–5,000 live births and is slightly more common in males. The defect may occur alone or may be associated with tracheoesophageal fistula, esophageal atresia, cardiac defects, or spinal or vertebral anomalies. Approximately 50% of children with intermediate or high imperforate anus will have long-term problems related to soiling, incontinence, or constipation. Many children with repaired low defects have constipation.

Risk Factors
No risk factors have been identified.

Prevention and Screening
There is no prevention. Screening for physical signs is done on all newborns.

Assessment
History
- No specific history

Physical Exam
- Absent or very small anal opening
- Absence of meconium or presence in urine
- Abdominal distention
- Flat perineum
- Absence of midline intergluteal groove

Diagnostic Studies
- Abdominal and pelvic ultrasound show malformation
- IV pyelogram and voiding cystourethrogram may show contact with urinary system
- MRI
- Radiography

Management
Invasive
- Surgical creation of an anal opening
- Depending on severity, a temporary colostomy
- Closure of fistulas
- Anoplasty, attaching the rectum to the created anus

Nonpharmacologic
- Manual dilation with a metallic dilator
- Enemas to prevent constipation
- Bowel training program for continued bowel incontinence
    - Daily bowel irrigations
    - Diet modification, fiber
    - Stool softeners

Pharmacologic
- Intravenous fluids to maintain fluid and electrolyte balance
- Pain management

Patient/Family Education
- Explanation of defect, surgery, treatment plan, possible complications
- Diagnostic tests
- Postoperative pain management
- Care of wound and peritoneum
- Colostomy care
- Manual dilation and enema administration
- Bowel training strategies

Outcomes and Follow-Up
- Child will not experience complications such as anal stricture or long-term bowel incontinence.
- Child will have normal bowel pattern without soilage or incontinence.
- Family will verbalize understanding of defect and treatment plan.
- Family will demonstrate care of wound, perineum, and colostomy.
- Family will demonstrate manual dilation and enema administration.
- Family will verbalize understanding of bowel training program.

PYLORIC STENOSIS

Description
Pyloric stenosis is a narrowing and lengthening of the pyloric canal between the stomach and the duodenum that usually develops in the first several weeks of life.

Etiology
The exact cause is unknown. The pylorus muscle becomes thickened, resulting in progressive narrowing and lengthening of the pyloric canal causing outlet obstruction.

Incidence and Demographics
The incidence is approximately 1 in 500 live births. It is more common in males and Whites, but rare in Asians.

Risk Factors
Infant with affected parent

Prevention and Screening
No prevention identified. Screening consists of evaluation of physical signs.

Assessment
History
- Vomiting without bile after feeding, which progresses in frequency and becomes projectile
- Hunger and irritability
- Weight loss

Physical Exam
- Hard, mobile, nontender, olive-shaped mass just right of umbilicus
- Visible peristaltic waves moving from left to right
- Signs of dehydration

Diagnostic Studies
- Ultrasound will show the enlarged pylorus
- Radiography will show gastric distention
- Upper GI will demonstrate delayed gastric emptying and narrow pyloric channel
- Blood studies may show metabolic alkalosis that becomes acidosis as dehydration progresses

Management
Invasive
- Laparoscopic pyloromyotomy, longitudinal incision of the pylorus to allow bulge and relieve obstruction

Nonpharmacologic
- Possibly nasogastric tube before surgery
- Gradual progression of feeding after surgery
- Frequent burping

Pharmacologic
- Preoperative and postoperative intravenous therapy to correct fluid and electrolyte imbalances
- Pain management

Patient/Family Education
- Explanation of defect and treatment plan
- Feeding progression
- Pain management
- Some postoperative vomiting is expected for 24–48 hours

Outcomes and Follow-Up

- The child's fluid and electrolyte balance will be restored before surgery.
- The child's incision site will show evidence of healing without infection.
- The child will experience effective pain management.
- The child will show no signs of dehydration.
- The child will regain lost weight and demonstrate adequate growth.
- The family will verbalize understanding of defect, treatment plan, feeding progression, and pain management.

GASTROESOPHAGEAL REFLUX

Description
Gastroesophageal reflux (GER) is the passage of gastric contents into the esophagus. Gastroesophageal reflux disease (GERD) involves gastroesophageal reflux with signs of esophagitis.

Etiology
Gastroesophageal reflux occurs when the lower esophageal sphincter relaxes or when the sphincter tone does not respond to changes in abdominal pressure, allowing gastric contents to pass into the esophagus or the oropharynx.

Incidence and Demographics
Gastroesophageal reflux peaks at approximately 4 months of age, with up to 40% of infants regurgitating more than half of their meals on a daily basis. The majority of these infants outgrow this by 12–15 months. About 5%–10% of older children complain about reflux symptoms on a weekly basis.

Risk Factors
- Familial history
- Obesity
- High-fat diet
- Eating quickly
- Smoke exposure may increase acid reflux in infants with wheezing or apparent life-threatening events
- Marked developmental delay

- Cerebral palsy
- Esophageal atresia
- Cystic fibrosis
- Bronchopulmonary dysplasia

Prevention and Screening

Prevention in infants includes avoidance of overfeeding. For older children, weight control and healthy diet are important. Screening consists of feeding history, pattern of vomiting, past medical history, family history, and growth measurements.

Assessment

History

- Risk factors
- Physical signs

Physical Exam

- Infants
- Feeding refusal
- Arching
- Irritability
- Recurrent regurgitation
- Poor weight gain
- Apnea or apparent life-threatening event (ALTE)

Older Children

- Heartburn
- Dysphagia or feeding refusal
- Recurrent vomiting
- Esophagitis
- Asthma
- Recurrent pneumonia
- Upper airway symptoms

Diagnostic Studies

- Upper gastrointestinal radiography may show delayed gastric emptying
- Esophageal pH monitoring to detect episodes of acidic reflux
- Multiple intraluminal electrical impedance measurement shows acidic and nonacidic reflux and associated respiratory symptoms
- Nuclear medicine scintigraphy shows both forms of reflux, gastric emptying, and possibly aspiration

Management

Invasive

- Nissen fundoplication antireflux surgery if nonpharmacologic management is unsuccessful
- Proximal portion of stomach wrapped around esophagus
- Recreates lower esophageal sphincter to prevent reflux

Nonpharmacologic

INFANTS
- Smaller, more frequent feeding
- Thickening formula with dry rice cereal decreases regurgitation and crying, but not intra-esophageal acid reflux
- Prethickened formula has similar effects
- Elevate head for 30 minutes after eating
- Prone position after feeding for infants who are awake
- Supine position for all sleeping infants to decrease risk for sudden infant death syndrome

OLDER CHILDREN
- Healthy diet
- Weight control
- Elevate head of bed
- Avoid smoking and alcohol
- Avoid nonsteroidal anti-inflammatory drugs (NSAIDs)

Pharmacologic

HISTAMINE2 RECEPTOR ANTAGONISTS (H2RAS)
- Ranitidine (Zantac)
- Famotidine (Pepcid)
- Cimetidine (Tagamet)

PROKINETICS
- Metoclopramide (Reglan)
- Bethanechol (Urecholine)
- Erythromycin

PROTEIN PUMP INHIBITORS (PPIS)
- Lansoprazole (Prevacid)
- Omeprazole (Prilosec)

Patient/Family Education
- Treatment plan
- Nonpharmacologic management
- Medication administration

Outcomes and Follow-Up
- Child will not experience further symptoms.
- Child will not experience complications such as esophagitis, peptic stricture, delayed growth, dental caries, recurrent otitis media, pneumonia, asthma, changes to lining of esophagus, or esophageal cancer.
- Family will verbalize understanding of treatment plan, nonpharmacologic management, and medication administration.

HERNIA

Description
A hernia is a protrusion of an organ or organs through an opening. The opening is in the diaphragm in congenital diaphragmatic hernia (CDH), through the umbilical ring in umbilical hernia, and through the processus vaginalis in males and through the round ligament in females in inguinal hernia.

Etiology
- Congenital diaphragmatic hernia happens at 8–10 weeks gestation with incomplete fusion of the diaphragm, resulting in protrusion of abdominal contents into the chest cavity causing compression and hypoplasia of the lung
- Umbilical hernia is due to opening of abdominal muscle at the umbilicus
- Inguinal hernias occur during the eighth month of gestation when the structures fail to close

Incidence and Demographics
- Congenital diaphragmatic hernias have a reported incidence of 1 in every 2,000 to 4,000 live births, and occur more frequently in males
- Umbilical hernias are more commonly occurring hernias and have an increased incidence in Blacks
- Inguinal hernias occur in 1%–4% of the population, more often in males, and more often on the right side

Risk Factors
- Prematurity
- Ventriculoperitoneal shunts
- Peritoneal dialysis
- Cystic fibrosis
- Hypospadias

Prevention and Screening
No prevention has been identified; screening for CDH is prenatal ultrasound

Assessment
History
- Prenatal polyhydramnios with CDH
- Bulge at umbilicus with crying or straining

Physical Exam
- Congenital diaphragmatic hernia
  - Cyanosis with severe respiratory distress
  - Absent breath sounds on affected side
- Umbilical hernia presents as an umbilical bulge that enlarges with crying or straining
- Inguinal hernia
  - Painless bulge in the scrotum or the labia that may be reduced into the peritoneal cavity
  - If the hernia is incarcerated, not reducible, the testicle or the intestine may become ischemic

Diagnostic Studies
- Congenital diaphragmatic hernia may sometimes be seen on prenatal ultrasound
- Radiography
- Scrotal ultrasound

Management
Invasive
- Congenital diaphragmatic hernia
  - Possibly extracorporeal membrane oxygenation (ECMO)
  - A few medical centers do fetal surgery for CDH
  - Surgical repair of diaphragm moving abdominal contents into the abdominal cavity
- Umbilical hernia may be surgically corrected if it does not resolve spontaneously by age 3–5 years
- Inguinal hernia
  - Surgical correction due to risk of incarceration
  - Incarceration requires immediate surgical repair

Nonpharmacologic
CONGENITAL DIAPHRAGMATIC HERNIA
- Possibly intubation and ventilation
- Nasogastric tube to low continuous suction
- Arterial and central venous lines

UMBILICAL HERNIA
- Pressure dressing for 48 hours after surgical repair
- Avoid strenuous activity or play for 2–3 weeks after surgery

INGUINAL HERNIA
- Keep incision site clean and dry
- Avoid strenuous activity or play for 2–3 weeks

Pharmacologic
- Congenital diaphragmatic hernia
  - Sedation and paralysis
  - Intravenous therapy to maintain fluid and electrolyte balance
- Pain management after surgical procedures

Patient/Family Education
- Explanation of defect and treatment plan
- Signs of incarceration such as irritability, refusal to eat, vomiting
- Measures to reduce inguinal hernia
- Postoperative care

Outcomes and Follow-Up
- The child with CDH will maintain open airway and effective respirations.
- The child will not experience complication of CDH such as chronic lung disease, failure to thrive, gastroesophageal reflux, cognitive impairment, musculoskeletal deformities, or delayed developmental gross motor milestones.

- The child will receive prompt medical attention for incarceration.
- The child's incision site will heal without complications.
- The family will verbalize understanding of defect and treatment plan.
- The family will demonstrate hernia reduction.
- The family will identify signs of incarceration.
- The family will verbalize understanding of home care.

INTUSSUSCEPTION

Description
Intussusception is the prolapse of one portion of the intestine into the immediately adjacent distal portion. The most common site is the ileocecal valve.

Etiology
Intussusception may be caused by hypertrophy of intestinal tissue after a viral infection. When the invagination occurs, the mesentery is pulled into the lumen causing vascular compression. This compression may lead to inflammation, edema, necrosis, and perforation.

Incidence and Demographics
Intussusception is seen most frequently in children between 3 months and 5 years of age. Sixty percent occurs before age 1, with a peak occurrence at 6–11 months. The yearly incidence in the United States is about 56 in 100,000 children.

Risk Factors
- Intestinal polyp
- Intestinal lymphoma
- Meckel diverticulum
- Henoch-Schönlein purpura

Prevention and Screening
- No prevention or screening strategies have been identified.

Assessment
History
- Episodes of intermittent, colicky abdominal pain
- Vomiting
- Anorexia
- Weight loss
- Diarrhea or rectal bleeding
- Bloody, mucus stools ("currant jelly stools")

Physical Exam
- Abdominal distention with palpable sausage-shaped mass in right upper abdomen
- Lethargy

Diagnostic Studies

- Radiography shows minimal gas in the right abdomen and ascending colon
- Ultrasound and CT scan show alternating intestinal rings
- Contrast enema with fluoroscopic guidance may reduce intussusceptions, but is contraindicated if perforation is suspected

Management

Invasive

- If enema is unsuccessful or the bowel has perforated, manual reduction with resection of nonviable intestine is done. If the child passes a normal stool, surgery is cancelled.

Nonpharmacologic

- Reduction with enema by radiologist
- Air enemas have shown higher reduction rates
- Some sites use barium, saline, or water

Pharmacologic

- Intravenous therapy to maintain fluid and electrolyte balance
- Antibiotics to prevent infection or treat peritonitis
- Pain management

Patient/Family Education

- Explanation of defect and treatment plan
- Pain management
- Home care after surgery
- Possibility of recurrence

Outcomes and Follow-Up

- The child's intussusceptions will be reduced with enema.
- The child will not experience perforation, peritonitis, or recurrence.
- The child will experience effective pain management.
- The family will verbalize understanding of defect and treatment plan.
- The family will verbalize understanding of home care and possibility of recurrence.

GASTROENTERITIS

Description

Gastroenteritis is acute infectious diarrhea.

Etiology

Gastroenteritis is spread by fecal–oral route. Common bacterial causes are *Escherichia coli, Salmonella, Shigella, Campylobacter, Yersinia, Aeromonas, Clostridium difficile,* and *Staphylococcus aureus.* Viral agents include rotavirus, Norwalk virus, small and round viruses, adenovirus, pestivirus, astrovirus, calicivirus, and paravirus. *Giardia lamblia, Cryptosporidium, Isospora belli, Microsporida, Strongyloides,* and *Entamoeba histolytica* are parasitic causes.

Incidence and Demographics

Rotavirus is the most common cause of diarrhea in children under 5 years of age. Foodborne pathogens include *Escherichia coli*, *Salmonella*, *Yersinia*, *Campylobacter*, *Clostridium*, and *Staphylococcus*. Children may also contact *Salmonella*, *Yersinia*, and *Campylobacter* from pets such as dogs, cats, hamsters, turtles, and iguanas. In the United States, about 200,000 children are hospitalized for gastroenteritis each year.

Risk Factors

- Infancy
- Immunocompromised state
- Poor hygiene
- Poor sanitation
- Lack of clean water
- Lack of refrigeration
- Nutritional deficiency
- Crowded living conditions

Prevention and Screening

- Maintaining good hygiene
- Regular handwashing
- Thorough cooking of food
- Maintaining food at appropriate temperatures
- Healthy diet
- Rotavirus pentavalent vaccine (RotaTeq) at 2, 4, and 6 months of age

Assessment

History

- Diarrhea
- Vomiting
- Decreased urine output

Physical Exam

- Lethargy
- Dry mucous membranes
- Acute weight loss
- Dark, sunken eyes
- Lack of tearing
- Loss of skin elasticity
- Increased pulse rate
- Decreased capillary refill
- Fever
- Cold, mottled extremities
- Sunken fontanel
- Perianal irritation

Diagnostic Studies
- Stool culture to identify causative agent
- Urine specific gravity to identify dehydration
- Complete blood count, serum electrolytes, creatinine, blood urea nitrogen (BUN) to identify dehydration

Management
Invasive
- No invasive management indicated

Nonpharmacologic
- Oral rehydration therapy (Pedialyte®, Enfalyte®), starting with small amounts and increasing slowly over a 4-hour period
- Avoid plain water, homemade sugar solution, carbonated beverages, apple juice, Jell-O®, meat broth
- Continue breastfeeding
- If feedings are tolerated without vomiting, resume age-appropriate diet within 4 hours of rehydration

Pharmacologic
- Intravenous fluids to replace lost fluid and to maintain fluid and electrolyte balance
- Antibiotics for *Shigella*, *Campylobacter*, *Vibrio cholera*, and *Clostridium difficile*

Patient/Family Education
- Signs of dehydration
- Oral rehydration process
- Avoid over-the-counter medications for vomiting or diarrhea
- Strategies to prevent spread of infection
- Skin care

Outcomes and Follow-Up
- The child will exhibit no signs of dehydration.
- The child will stop vomiting and episodes of diarrhea will decrease.
- The child will maintain skin integrity.
- The family will verbalize understanding of signs of dehydration, treatment plan, infection prevention strategies, and skin care.

HIRSCHSPRUNG DISEASE

Description
Hirschsprung disease is the absence of ganglion nerve cells in the distal colon causing a functional bowel obstruction. The section of bowel proximal to the affected area becomes dilated; hence, the disorder is also called aganglionic megacolon. As the bowel distends, pressure on the bowel wall increases and blood flow decreases, leading to bacterial growth that can cause enterocolitis, inflammation of the intestine, and ulceration of the bowel wall.

Etiology

Hirschsprung disease is caused by failure of the ganglion cells to move through the neural crest during the fourth to twelfth weeks of gestation.

Incidence and Demographics

The incidence of Hirschsprung disease is 1 in 5,000 live births. The disease is limited to the rectosigmoid area in 80% of cases. Enterocolitis, with a 20% mortality rate, occurs most often in the second and third months of life. It is more common in males.

Risk Factors

No identified risk factors.

Prevention and Screening

No prevention. Screen newborns for passage of meconium and evaluate neonates' bowel patterns.

Assessment

History

- Failure to pass meconium until after the first 24 hours of life
- Chronic constipation

Physical Exam

- Bilious vomiting
- Abdominal distention
- Refusal to feed
- Liquid stool
- Signs of enterocolitis include abdominal distention, explosive diarrhea, fever, blood in the stool
- Children with short affected bowel segments may be diagnosed when older, exhibiting ribbon-like stools, abdominal distention, and failure to thrive

Diagnostic Studies

- Radiography may show dilated bowel
- Anorectal manometry shows absence of internal anal sphincter relaxation
- Rectal biopsy confirms diagnosis by showing absence of ganglion cells

Management

Invasive

- Surgical resection of the aganglionic bowel and anastomosis of the proximal normal bowel to the anal canal, called ileoanal pull-through anastomosis
- Possible surgical correction of anorectal stenosis, a common complication
- With enterocolitis or significantly dilated colon, colostomy to allow bowel to return to normal size
- Surgical pull-through 4 to 6 months after colostomy

Nonpharmacologic

PREOPERATIVE CARE
- Serial rectal irrigations to decompress and clean bowel
- Measurement of abdominal circumference

POSTOPERATIVE CARE
- Nasogastric tube to suction
- Intravenous fluids
- Wound care
- Colostomy care
- Avoid rectal medications and thermometers for 2–3 weeks
- Manual dilations for several months to prevent stricture

Pharmacologic
- Antibiotics to prevent or treat infection
- Pain management

Patient/Family Education
- Explanation of disease and treatment plan
- Wound care
- Colostomy care
- Manual dilation procedure
- Constipation prevention strategies, including high-fiber diet

Outcomes and Follow-Up
- The child will maintain normal fluid and electrolyte balance.
- The child will assume usual diet.
- The child will show signs of wound healing.
- The child will exhibit normal bowel patterns.
- The child will not experience complications such as incontinence or enterocolitis.
- The family will verbalize understanding of disease and treatment plan.
- The family will demonstrate wound care, colostomy care, and manual dilation.
- The family will verbalize understanding of constipation prevention.
- The family will verbalize signs of enterocolitis.

MALABSORPTION SYNDROMES

Description
Malabsorption syndromes are digestive disorders characterized by chronic diarrhea and impaired absorption of fluids and nutrients. Two common pediatric syndromes are celiac disease and short-bowel syndrome. Celiac disease, also called gluten-sensitive enteropathy or celiac sprue, is an autoimmune disorder with intestinal intolerance to dietary wheat gliadin and related proteins. Short-bowel syndrome (SBS) is a decrease in the mucosal surface area of the intestine.

Etiology

The child with celiac disease is unable to completely digest the protein gluten. The small intestine absorbs these proteins, causing an inflammatory reaction targeting the mucosa. Damage to the mucosa results in villous atrophy and decreased surface area for absorption of fluids and nutrients.

In children, short-bowel syndrome is usually caused by necrotizing enterocolitis, volvulus, jejunal atresias, and gastroschisis that require intestinal resection. Although rare, short-bowel syndrome may be congenital.

Incidence and Demographics

The incidence of celiac disease is 3–13 per 1,000 children. It is more prevalent in women and in Europe, but rarely seen in Asians or Blacks.

A loss of more than 70% of the small bowel results in severe malabsorption in SBS. Infants and children with SBS usually die from total parenteral nutrition (TPN) complications.

Risk Factors

Celiac Disease
- First-degree relative with the disease
- Down syndrome
- Rheumatoid arthritis
- Type 1 diabetes mellitus

Short-Bowel Syndrome
- Prematurity
- Bowel resection

Prevention and Screening
- No prevention or widespread screening indicated

Assessment

History

CELIAC DISEASE
- Constipation or diarrhea
- Flatulence
- Steatorrhea
- Failure to thrive
- Irritability
- Anorexia, nausea, vomiting
- Abdominal pain, distension, bloating

SBS
- Diarrhea
- Steatorrhea
- Fatigue
- Rectal bleeding

Physical Exam

CELIAC DISEASE

- Abdominal distention and pain
- Pallor
- Muscle wasting

SBS

- Pallor
- Failure to thrive

Diagnostic Studies

CELIAC DISEASE

- Serum immunoglobulin A (IgA)
- IgA tissue transglutaminase (tTG)
- Antiendomysium (EMA)
- Small bowel biopsy

SBS

- Blood studies: Anemia, iron deficiency
- Upper GI
- Colonoscopy

Management

Invasive

CELIAC DISEASE

- No invasive treatment indicated

SBS

- Intestinal surgical procedures and intestinal transplant have been used, but not accepted as routine care

Nonpharmacologic

CELIAC DISEASE

- Gluten-free diet: No wheat, rye, barley, and possibly oats (found extensively in processed food)
- Temporary lactose-free, low-fiber diet while bowel is inflamed

SBS

- Nonnutritive sucking, oral stimulation
- Small amounts of oral feeding

Pharmacologic

CELIAC DISEASE

- Iron, folic acid, and fat-soluble vitamin supplements as needed

SBS

- Initially, total parenteral nutrition (TPN) through a central line
- Gradual introduction of enteral nutrition of an easily absorbed formula
- Periodic antibiotics to prevent infection
- Vitamin supplements
- Histamine receptor antagonist medications for increased gastric acid
  - Ranitidine (Zantac)
  - Famotidine (Pepcid)
  - Cimetidine (Tagamet)

Patient/Family Education

CELIAC DISEASE

- Disease process
- Gluten-free diet
- Complications of noncompliance

SBS

- Disease and treatment plan
- Feeding management: TPN, enteral feeding
- Oral stimulation strategies
- Medication administration
- Signs of complications

Outcomes and Follow-Up

Celiac Disease

- The child will experience relief of symptoms with gluten-free diet.
- The child will demonstrate healing of intestinal mucosa with increased tolerance of lactose and fiber.
- The child will demonstrate adequate growth.
- The family will verbalize understanding of disease process.
- The family will identify sources of gluten and plan diet to meet nutritional needs.

Short-Bowel Syndrome

- The child will not experience complications of long-term TPN.
- The child's small intestine will increase mucosal surface area as evidenced by tolerance of enteral feedings.
- The child will demonstrate adequate growth.
- The family will verbalize understanding of disease process and treatment plan.
- The family will demonstrate management of central line and enteral feeding.
- The family will demonstrate effective medication administration.

INGESTIONS AND POISONINGS

Description
Accidental or unintentional ingestion of toxic substances is one of the most common pediatric emergencies.

Etiology
Young children ingest substances because of their normal developmental curiosity and experimentation, imitation behavior, and misidentification of substances that look like familiar beverages or candy. Another cause is therapeutic error resulting in medication overdose.

Incidence and Demographics
The peak age for poisoning is 1–3 years. In 2006, 38% of poison exposure involved children younger than 3 years of age and 51% occurred in children younger than 6. Children under 6 were involved in the majority of exposures, but comprised only 2.4% of verified fatalities. Common substances ingested are cosmetics and personal care products, cleaning substances, analgesics, foreign bodies, plants, topical preparations, cough and cold products, pesticides, vitamins, gastrointestinal preparations, antimicrobials, art and craft supplies, antihistamines, hormones, and hydrocarbons.

Risk Factors
- Access to toxic substances
- Lack of child-resistant medication containers
- Young developmental age
- History of previous ingestion
- Hyperactivity, rebelliousness, impulsivity, pica
- Environmental change or chaos
- Parental mental illness, depression, social isolation

Prevention and Screening
- Household products and medications stored in locked units out of child's sight and reach
- Store in original containers
- Child-resistant packaging
- Prevent child from seeing adult take medication
- Call it medication, not candy
- Teach children not to eat or drink anything that they cannot identify
- Evaluation of physical signs

Assessment
History
- History of ingestion or physical signs

Physical Exam
GASTROINTESTINAL SIGNS
- Abdominal pain
- Vomiting
- Diarrhea
- Anorexia
- Respiratory and circulatory signs

RESPIRATIONS MAY BE DEPRESSED, LABORED, SHALLOW, OR RAPID
- Skin may be cool, clammy, pale, or cyanotic
- Signs of shock
- Slow capillary refill
- Rapid, weak pulse
- Decreased blood pressure

CENTRAL NERVOUS SYSTEM SIGNS
- Seizures
- Overstimulation or lethargy
- Dizziness
- Loss of consciousness
- Coma

SIGNS OF CORROSIVE INGESTION
- Edema of the lips, tongue, or pharynx
- White or ulcerated mucosa
- Burning in mouth, throat, or stomach
- Vomiting
- Blood in saliva
- Drooling
- Agitation

SIGNS OF SHOCK
- Signs of hydrocarbon ingestion
- Nausea and vomiting
- Coughing, gagging
- Weakness
- Lethargy
- Respiratory distress

Diagnostic Studies
- Toxicology screening of blood or urine

Management
Invasive
- Hemodialysis and hemofiltration in severe cases

Nonpharmacologic
- Intubation for child without adequate gag reflex or altered mental status
- Gastric lavage unless child has unprotected airway, altered mental status, or ingested a corrosive substance
- Whole-bowel irrigation without contraindications noted in item above
- Cardiac monitoring

Pharmacologic
- Activated charcoal unless child has unprotected airway, altered mental status, altered bowel function, caustic ingestion, hydrocarbon ingestion, foreign body ingestion
- Urinary alkalinization with intravenous sodium bicarbonate to enhance renal excretion of weakly acidic drugs
- Specific antidotes such as N-acetylcysteine (Mucomyst) for acetaminophen or naloxone of opioids
- Intravenous fluids to maintain fluid and electrolyte balance

Patient/Family Education
- Prevention strategies
- Developmental risk factors
- Medication dosing guidelines
- Physical signs of poisoning
- Phone number of local poison control center

Outcomes and Follow-Up
- The child will recover without complications.
- The child will verbalize understanding of poison prevention strategies.
- The child will not have future access to toxic substances.
- The child will not experience additional ingestions.
- The family will verbalize understanding of treatment plan.
- The family will verbalize understanding of prevention strategies.
- The family will identify hazards in the home.
- The family will take steps to poison-proof the home.
- The family will identify physical signs of poisoning.
- The family will post the number of the local poison control center near their telephone.

APPENDICITIS

Description
Inflammation of the vermiform appendix

Etiology
Appendicitis results when the lumen of the appendix is obstructed by fecalith (hardened stool), microorganisms, or parasites. The obstruction causes mucus to increase pressure in the lumen, leading to compression of the blood vessels with progressive inflammation. The process can progress to gangrenous appendicitis. A ruptured or perforated appendix can cause progressive peritonitis.

Incidence and Demographics
78,000, approximately 1%, children younger than 15 years of age were hospitalized for appendicitis in 2005. The peak incidence is 10–12 years of age. It is uncommon in children younger than 2 years.

Risk Factors

No risk factors have been definitively identified, although individuals consuming diets high in sugars and low in fiber have shown increased incidence of appendicitis.

Prevention and Screening

No prevention has been identified. Children experiencing signs of appendicitis should be evaluated by a surgeon.

Assessment

History
- Child may have experienced nausea, vomiting, fever, abdominal pain

Physical Exam
- Vomiting
- Rectal tenderness
- Rebound tenderness
- Fever
- Psoas sign: Pain in the right hip
- Pain migrating from the umbilicus to right lower quadrant

Diagnostic Studies
- Elevated white blood cell count and elevated band cells
- CT scan or ultrasound
- Common organisms are *Escherichia coli* and *Klebsiella*
- Urinalysis to rule out urinary tract infection

Management

Invasive
- Appendectomy, the surgical removal of appendix via open or laparoscopic incision
- Possible drain placement for peritonitis

Nonpharmacologic
- Position for comfort
- Progressive ambulation with small pillow to support incision site
- Advance diet as tolerated
- Possible nasogastric tube for ruptured or gangrenous appendix
- Care of incision

Pharmacologic
- IV fluids to maintain fluid and electrolyte balance
- Pain management
- Antibiotics to prevent or treat infections

Patient/Family Education
- Diagnostic tests, disease process
- Preparation for surgery
- Postoperative care including ambulation, diet, pain management
- Home care, including activity, care of incision, reasons to call healthcare provider

Outcomes and Follow-Up
- Child and family will verbalize understanding of preoperative, postoperative, and home care.
- The child will experience effective pain control.
- The child will show no signs of infection.
- The child will show evidence of wound healing.
- The child will show evidence of adequate hydration and return to usual diet.

INFLAMMATORY BOWEL DISEASE

Description
Inflammatory bowel disease (IBD) is chronic inflammation of the intestine. The most common forms are ulcerative colitis (UC) and Crohn's disease (CD). UC affects the colon while CD may involve the entire gastrointestinal tract, but most commonly the ileum.

Etiology
IBD is an immune disease. The immune system reacts to antigens in bacteria or in food, causing an inflammatory process. In IBD, the intestinal mucosa becomes inflamed with ulceration, bleeding, edema, and decreased absorption of fluid and electrolytes.

Incidence and Demographics
- The incidence of ulcerative colitis is 3.5 new cases per 100,000 per year; incidence of Crohn's disease is 3.11 per 100,000
- Average age of onset for ulcerative colitis is 12–20 years of age; for Crohn's disease, 15–25 years of age
- IBD is more prevalent in people from higher socioeconomic levels and living in urban areas and in Whites

Risk Factors
- Family history

Prevention and Screening
- No prevention has been identified and screening involves evaluation of physical signs

Assessment
History
ULCERATIVE COLITIS
- Abdominal pain, cramping
- Bloody diarrhea
- Painful stooling
- Mucous in stool
- Anorexia

CROHN'S DISEASE
- Abdominal pain, cramping
- Diarrhea
- Weight loss
- Nausea
- Burning epigastric pain
- Anorexia

Physical Exam
ULCERATIVE COLITIS
- Growth failure
- Joint pain
- Rash

CROHN'S DISEASE
- Fever
- Rash
- Joint pain
- Lymphadenopathy
- Growth failure
- Perianal skin tags, abscesses, fissures, fistulas
- Mouth ulcers
- Inflammation of the iris, ciliary body, or choroid

Diagnostic Studies
- CBC to assess for anemia
- Elevated white blood cell count with Crohn's disease
- Elevated erythrocyte sedimentation rate
- Elevated circulating perinuclear antineutrophil cytoplasmic antibody (pANCA)
- Upper GI
- Endoscopy with biopsy
- Colonoscopy

Management
Invasive
- If unresponsive to pharmacologic treatment, surgical removal of the colon or part of the small intestine with ileostomy or pull-through
- Surgical treatment for complications of Crohn's disease including abscess, bowel obstruction, or fistulas between the intestine and skin

Nonpharmacologic
- Healthy diet, including increased fruits, vegetables, water
- Decreased intake of sweetened beverages
- Smaller, more frequent meals
- Identify foods that increase symptoms
- Avoid high-fiber foods such as seeds, popcorn, corn
- Possibly enteral or parenteral nutrition

Pharmacologic
- Corticosteroids
  - Prednisone
  - Methylprednisolone (Solu-Medrol)
  - Budesonide (Pulmicort)
- Anti-inflammatory medications
  - Sulfasalazine (Azulfidine)
  - Olsalazine (Dipentum)
- Nonspecific immunosuppressives
  - Azathioprine (Imuran, Azasan)
  - Mercaptopurine
- Monoclonal antibodies
  - Infliximab
  - Adalimumab
  - Natalizumab
- Antibiotics for infection
  - Metronidazole (Flagyl)
  - Ciprofloxacin (Cipro)
- Vitamins, minerals, nutritional supplements for specific deficiencies

Patient/Family Education
- Disease process
- Treatment plan
- Nonpharmacologic management
- Medication administration

Outcomes and Follow-Up
- The child will experience relief of diarrhea, rectal bleeding, and abdominal pain.
- The child will display adequate growth.
- The child and family will verbalize understanding of disease, treatment plan, nonpharmacologic management, and medication administration.
- The child and family will identify foods that aggravate symptoms.

REFERENCES

Allen, P. L. (2004). Guidelines for the diagnosis and treatment of celiac disease in children. *Pediatric Nursing, 30,* 473–476.

Applegate, K. E. (2008). Intussusception in children: Imaging choices. *Seminars in Roentgenology, 43,* 15–19.

Bronstein, A. C., Spyker, D. A., Cantilena, L. R., Green, J., Rumack, B. H., & Heard, S. E. (2007). 2006 annual report of the American association of poison control centers' national poison data system. *Clinical Toxicology, 45,* 815–917.

Carmichael, S. L., Shaw, G. M., Ma, C., Werler, M. M., Rasmussen, S. A., & Lammer, E. J. (2007). Maternal corticosteroid use and orofacial clefts. *American Journal of Obstetrics & Gynecology, 197,* 585.e1–585.e7.

Doody, D. P. (2006). Anorectal anomalies: A review of surgeries past. *Seminars in Colon & Rectal Surgery, 17,* 3–9.

Ebell, M. H. (2008). Diagnosis of appendicitis: Part I. History and physical examination. *American Family Physician, 77,* 828–830.

Ebell, M. H. (2008). Diagnosis of appendicitis: Part II. Laboratory and imaging tests. *American Family Physician, 77,* 1153–1155.

Hasosah, M., Lemberg, D. A., Skarsgard, E., & Schreiber, R. (2008). Congenital short bowel syndrome: A case report and review of the literature. *The Canadian Journal of Gastroenterology, 22,* 71–74.

Hill, K. D., & Hill, I. D. (2005). Celiac disease: Fundamentals for pediatricians. *Contemporary Pediatrics.* Retrieved from http://www.skyscape.com/Content:Celiacdisease

Hockenberry, M. J., & Wilson, D. (2007). *Wong's nursing care of infants and children.* St. Louis, MO: Mosby Elsevier.

Jackson, C. S., & Buchman, A. L. (2004). The nutritional management of short bowel syndrome. *Nutrition in Clinical Care, 7,* 114–121.

Kasten, E. F., Schmidt, S. P., Zickler, C. F., Berner, E., Damian, L. K., Christian, G. M., et al. (2008). Team care of the patient with cleft lip and palate. *Current Problems in Pediatric and Adolescent Health Care, 5,* 138–158.

Kessmann, J. (2006). Hirschsprung's disease: Diagnosis and management. *American Family Physician, 74,* 1319–1322.

Koslap-Petraco, M. B. (2006). Homecare issues in rotavirus gastroenteritis. *Journal of the American Academy of Nurse Practitioners, 18,* 422–428.

Kovesi, T., & Rubin, S. (2004). Long-term complications of congenital esophageal atresia and/or tracheoesophageal fistula. *Chest, 126,* 915–925.

Marcus, K. A., Halbertsma, F. J. J., & Severijnen, R. S. V. M. (2008). Presentation of congenital diaphragmatic hernia after the neonatal period. *Clinical Pediatrics, 47,* 171–175.

McCollough, M., & Sharieff, G. Q. (2006). Abdominal pain in children. *Pediatric Clinics of North America, 53,* 107–137.

Nisell, M., Ojmyr-Joelsson, M., Frenckner, B., Rydelius, P., & Christensson, K. (2003). How a family is affected when a child is born with anorectal malformation. Interviews with three patients and their parents. *International Pediatric Nursing, 18,* 423–432.

Orenstein, S. R., & McGowan, J. D. (2008). Efficacy of conservative therapy as taught in the primary care setting for symptoms suggesting infant gastroesophageal reflux. *The Journal of Pediatrics, 152,* 310–314.

Presutti, R. J., Cangemi, J. R., Cassidy, H. D., & Hill, D. A. (2007). Celiac disease. *American Family Physician, 76,* 1795–1802.

Puckett, B. (2006). Congenital diaphragmatic hernia: Two case studies with atypical presentations. *Neonatal Network, 25,* 239–249.

Pulsifer, A. (2005). Pediatric genitourinary examination: A clinician's reference. *Urologic Nursing, 25,* 163–168.

Robertson, J., & Shilkofski, N. (Eds.). (2005). *The Harriet Lane handbook.* Philadelphia: Mosby.

Shatsky, M. (2006). Rotavirus vaccine, live, oral, pentavalent (RotaTeq) for prevention of rotavirus gastroenteritis. *American Family Physician, 74,* 1014–1015.

Sherman, P. M., Gold, B. D., Harnsberger, J. K., & Czinn, S. J. (2004). *Sharing solutions in pediatric gastroenterology: Building algorithms for gastroesophageal reflux disease.* Retrieved from http://www.medscape.com/viewarticle/494079_1

Simpson, T., & Ivey, J. (2007). Stomach pain. *Pediatric Nursing, 33,* 136–137.

Tesselaar, C. K., Postema, R. R., van Dooren, M. F., Allegaert, K., & Tibboel, D. (2004). Congenital diaphragmatic hernia and situs inversus totalis. *Pediatrics, 113,* 256–258.

Tobias, N., Mason, D., Lutkenhoff, M., Stoops, M., & Ferguson, D. (2008). Management principles of organic causes of childhood constipation. *Journal of Pediatric Health Care, 22,* 12–23.

Torpy, J. M., Lynm, C., & Glass, R. M. (2008). Crohn disease. *Journal of the American Medical Association, 299,* 1738.

Vieira, A. R. (2008). Unraveling human cleft lip and palate research. *Journal of Dental Research, 87,* 119–125.

Wilkerson, R., Northington, L., & Fisher, W. (2005). Ingestion of toxic substances by infants and children: What we don't know can hurt. *Critical Care Nurse, 25*(4), 35–44.

Winter, H. S., Gold, B. D., & Nelson, S. P. (2005). *Pediatric GERD: A problem-based approach to understanding treatment.* Retrieved from http://medscape.com/viewarticle/517267

Yaffe, S. J., & Aranda, J. V. (2005). *Neonatal and pediatric pharmacology: Therapeutic principles in practice.* Philadelphia: Lippincott, Williams, and Wilkins.

12

Genitourinary Disorders

Karen Corlett, MSN, RN-BC, CPNP-AC/PC, PNP-BC

HYPOSPADIUS

Description
Abnormal positioning of the male urethra on the underside of the penis. Severity varies from mild malposition to urethral opening at base of penis.

Etiology
- Likely multifactorial
- Familial predisposition
- Endocrine abnormalities
- Genetic and environmental influences not yet clearly identified

Incidence and Demographics
- 0.7% of live-born males affected
- Most common in Whites, rare in Hispanic populations

Risk Factors
- Family history
- Disorders of testosterone production or sensitivity

Prevention and Screening
- No prevention or screening indicated

Assessment
- Inspection of the penis and urethra
  - Ventral location of urethra
    - Positioned low or on underside of the penis
  - May have "bend" in penis due to chordee
  - Incomplete or redundant foreskin
- Downward urinary stream
- Check for normal position of testes
- Evaluate for inguinal hernia
- Family's understanding of problem and plans for correction
  - Psychosocial support for child and family

Management
- Do not circumcise
  - Foreskin may be useful in surgical repair
- Testosterone treatment preoperatively
  - To augment penile growth in some patients
- Surgical repair
  - Before 18 months of age
  - Elongate, repair, and reposition urethra
  - Repair chordee
  - Restore structure and function
- Postoperative care
  - Foley catheter to avoid urethral scarring
    - Adequate fluids to promote good urine output (UOP)
  - Dressing maintenance or changes as ordered
  - Pain management
  - Infection prevention or early identification

Outcomes and Follow-Up
- Discharge teaching
  - Dressing maintenance or changes
    - Antibiotic ointments or creams as prescribed
  - Fluids to maintain good UOP
  - Urethral catheter care if discharged with catheter in place
  - Signs and symptoms of infection
  - Pain management
- Return for follow-up evaluation, dressing change, and/or catheter removal

- Psychosocial support for child
  - Child life services
- Potential complications
  - Urethral strictures
  - Urethral fistulas
  - Retraction of urethra away from surgically repositioned site
  - Surgical site or urinary tract infection

VESICOURETURAL REFLUX (VUR)

Description
Backward flow of urine within the urinary tract, from bladder to ureter and at times back into kidney.

Etiology
- Failure of one-way valve mechanism of ureters as they enter the bladder wall
  - Faulty valve
  - Abnormal position of valve
- Can be transient occurrence during urinary tract infection (UTI)

Incidence and Demographics
- True incidence unknown because not all children screened
- Most common anatomic abnormality affecting the urinary tract
- Diagnosed in up to 30% of children who have had a UTI

Risk Factors
- Parent with VUR
- Sibling with VUR

Prevention and Screening
- No prevention or screening indicated

Assessment
- Most patients asymptomatic
- Routine screening post-UTI
  - Voiding cystourethrogram or cystogram
- Severity graded from I (mild) to V (severe)

Management
- Education for child and family
  - Disease process
  - Signs and symptoms of urinary tract infection
    - Potential for permanent kidney damage
  - Importance of continued follow-up

- Dependent upon severity of VUR
  - Mild cases may resolve with somatic and ureteral growth
  - Careful monitoring for urinary tract infection
  - Prevention of renal scarring and permanent injury
- Medications
  - Antibiotic prophylaxis
  - Anticholinergics to decrease bladder pressure
- Surgery
  - For medical treatment failures
    - Recurrent UTIs or progressive kidney damage
  - Repositioning of ureters in bladder wall
  - Urinary diversion away from bladder wall if unable to achieve competent valves with repositioning
- Postoperative care
  - Meticulous attention to all portals and devices providing urinary drainage
    - Stents, catheters, diversionary drains
    - Patency of devices
    - Infection control measures
  - Patient and family education
    - Care and patency of stents, drainage tubes, or diversion devices
    - Signs and symptoms of infection
    - Importance of adequate fluid intake to maintain urine flow

URINARY TRACT INFECTIONS

Description
- Infection of the urinary tract
- Urethritis
  - Urethral infection
- Cystitis
  - Bladder infection
- Pyelonephritis
  - Infection of the kidney

Etiology
- Bacteria enter urinary tract and cause infection
- Enter via bloodstream
  - Most common in infants
- Ascending route via urethra
- Structural anomalies
  - Causing stasis, obstruction, or reflux
- Bacteria
  - *Escherichia coli* most common
  - *Klebsiella pneumoniae, Enterobacter, Pseudomonas*
    - More common in those with anatomic abnormalities

Incidence and Demographics
- 1% of newborns
- Girls > boys outside of newborn period
  - Uncircumcised males have slightly higher incidence

Risk Factors
- Female (shorter urethra)
- Anatomic abnormalities

Prevention and Screening
- No prevention or screening indicated

Assessment
- Signs and symptoms of urinary tract infection
  - May be vague, especially in infants
  - Fever, chills, and back pain for pyelonephritis
  - Dysuria
    - Frequency, urgency, burning, itching
  - Vomiting, nausea, diarrhea, anorexia
  - Irritability, fussiness in infants
- Urinalysis with culture and sensitivity
  - Done before initiation of antibiotics
  - Catheter specimen is gold standard for culture
    - Clean-catch midstream urine in cooperative older children
    - Bagged specimen in young children may be used
      - Risk of contamination by skin flora
  - Bacteria and white blood cells on urinalysis
  - Identification of bacteria on culture
- May draw blood culture in infants due to risk of infection from or spread to bloodstream

Management
- Antibiotics for suspected infection
  - Tailor or narrow spectrum once organism known
  - Most infections treated as outpatients
    - Hospitalization and intravenous antibiotics for infants or those with symptoms of systemic illness
- Documentation of sterile urine posttreatment
- Evaluation of urinary tract for anomalies once infection cleared
- Education for patient and family
  - Signs and symptoms of worsening illness
  - Signs and symptoms of recurrent UTI
  - Importance of full antibiotic course as prescribed
  - Importance of follow-up for clearance and potential cause of infection

ACUTE GLOMERULONEPHRITIS

Description
Acute inflammation of the renal glomeruli. Glomeruli are the tufts of capillaries responsible for filtration of blood/plasma into the kidney. Inflammation affects filtration and impacts renal function. Permanent scarring can occur.

Etiology
- Postinfectious
  - Group A beta-hemolytic streptococcus
  - Immune mediated postinfectious illness
- Direct damage to glomeruli from renal or systemic disease

Incidence and Demographics
- Incidence is unknown
- Highest incidence in preschoolers and school age children
- Boys > girls

Risk Factors
- History of Group A beta-hemolytic streptococcal infection
- Renal disease

Assessment
- Urinalysis, urine culture, serum electrolytes, blood urea nitrogen (BUN) and creatinine
- Symptoms:
  - Protein and blood in the urine
  - Low serum albumin levels
  - Edema
    - Periorbital and dependent
  - Hypertension
    - Frequent monitoring
  - Low urine output
  - Elevated creatinine
  - Electrolyte abnormalities
    - High potassium most concerning
  - Fatigue, anorexia
- History of streptococcal infection
  - Throat culture
- History or identification of kidney abnormality
  - Renal biopsy
- Elevated serum complement

Management

- Treat symptoms
  - Diuretics
  - Antihypertensives
  - Monitoring of intake vs. output, daily weights
  - Close monitoring of electrolytes, BUN, and creatinine
  - Dietary restrictions as ordered
    - Limitation of sodium, potassium, protein, phosphorous, and/or fluid intake
- Dialysis for renal failure not manageable with above treatments
- Education of patient and family
  - Signs and symptoms of worsening renal failure
    - Worsening edema, blood in urine, marked increase or decrease in urine output
    - Altered mental status
    - Laboratory abnormalities
      - Hyperkalemia
      - Rising BUN and/or creatinine
  - Medications
    - Antihypertensives and/or diuretics
    - Binders to absorb electrolytes
      - Kayexalate
      - Phosphate binders
  - Fluid and/or dietary restrictions
  - Importance of continued follow-up until resolution

Outcomes and Follow-Up

- Most children recover fully in 1–3 weeks
- Some progress to chronic renal failure
  - Immediate or over long term
- Routine specialty follow-up if residual disease

NEPHROTIC SYNDROME

Description

Renal disease characterized by massive protein in the urine, resultant low serum albumin, and diffuse edema.

Etiology

- Often unknown
- Scarring or disease of the glomeruli
- Congenital nephropathy

Incidence and Demographics

- Incidence in children unknown
- Most frequent in children 1–5 years old
- Boys > girls

Risk Factors
- Glomerular scarring, abnormality, or inflammation
- Congenital nephrotic syndrome

Assessment
- Urine studies
  - For protein and glomerular filtration rate
  - Record of intake vs. output
- Serum studies
  - Electrolytes, BUN, creatinine
  - Albumin and other proteins (hemoglobin, platelets, immunoglobulins)
  - Complement is low
- Blood pressure monitoring
- Daily weights, evaluation of edema
- Renal biopsy may be indicated to delineate cause

Management
- Corticosteroids
  - Decrease inflammation and protein loss
  - 1–2 month duration with taper
  - Relapse of proteinuria frequent
    - Treated with short steroid burst
  - Patient and family education of side effects
    - Immunosuppression and increased risk of infection
    - Increased appetite, weight gain, unusual distribution of weight gain
    - Thinning of skin and bones
- Albumin replacement
- Electrolyte monitoring and management
- Diuretics for severe edema
  - Intake vs. output
  - Overall urine output
- Dietary restrictions
  - Sodium most frequent limitation
- Antihypertensives as ordered
- Meticulous skin hygiene
- Infection surveillance, prompt treatment
- Serum glucose monitoring
  - Glucose effects of steroid therapy
- Other immune suppressants may be used if steroids fail to achieve remission
- Dialysis if renal failure

Outcomes and Follow-Up
- Close monitoring of urine protein as indicator of relapse
  - Teach patient/family home urine dipstick testing
- Daily weights by family postdischarge

- Medication teaching
  - Steroids as above
    - Hand hygiene and avoidance of sick contacts
  - Antihypertensives
    - Home blood pressure monitoring can be challenging in the young
    - Procurement of appropriate medical devices for monitoring
- Dietary/nutritional counseling
- High rate of relapse requiring reinstitution of steroids
- May progress to renal failure

WILMS TUMOR

Description
- Malignant tumor of the kidney
- Also referred to as nephroblastoma

Etiology and Risk Factors
- Most cases without cause or genetic link
- Some familial predisposition
  - Genetic markers identified
  - Autosomal dominant transmission
- Associated syndromes:
  - Beckwith-Wiedemann syndrome
  - Denys-Drash syndrome
  - WAGR syndrome
- Associated findings:
  - Aniridia
  - Hemihypertrophy
  - Neurofibromatosis
  - Genitourinary anomalies

Incidence and Demographics
- ~8 per million children
- Most common in 2–5-year-olds

Prevention and Screening
No prevention or screening indicated

Assessment
- Painless abdominal mass in otherwise healthy child
- Ultrasound of mass
  - Unilateral or bilateral kidney involvement
- Blood work to evaluate kidney function, electrolytes, hematological system
- Chest x-ray and chest CT scan to evaluate for metastases
- Surgical biopsy
  - Excision as well

Management
- Do not palpate mass
  - Risk of rupture of encapsulated tumor and spread of cancerous cells
- Surgical resection of tumor
  - Entire kidney may be removed
  - Challenging if both kidneys involved
  - Most affected kidney is removed
- Postoperative care
  - Pain management
  - Monitoring and treatment of hypertension
  - Prevention or early identification of infection
  - Careful documentation of fluid and electrolyte balance
  - Lab studies to follow function of remaining kidney
  - Patient and family education as to disease process and treatment plan
- Chemotherapy is routine
- Radiation only if recurrence or incomplete surgical removal

Outcomes and Follow-Up
- Overall survival rate > 90%
- At risk for recurrence of nephroblastoma
- Continued surveillance of kidney function
  - No contact sports due to risk of injury to remaining kidney
- Follow-up for short- and long-term side effects of chemotherapy
- At increased risk of additional cancers later in life

SEXUALLY TRANSMITTED INFECTIONS (STIs)

Description, Etiology, Incidence, and Demographics
Infections passed from person to person through sexual intercourse or genital contact

Chlamydia
- Centers for Disease Control and Prevention (CDC) received > 1 million reports of *Chlamydia* infection in 2006
- Caused by *Chlamydia trachomatis*
- Abnormal vaginal or penile discharge
- Burning on urination
- Many without symptoms

Genital Herpes
- CDC estimates 45 million people age 12 and older have had genital herpes
- Caused by herpes simplex virus type 1 or 2
- Painful blisters on genitals
  - First outbreak may have systemic illness as well
- Recurrent outbreaks common but shorter and less severe
  - Itching, burning, or tingling may precede outbreak

Genital Warts
- CDC estimates 20 million Americans currently infected with human papillomavirus (HPV) and > 6 million new cases/year
- Caused by a variety of different human papillomaviruses
- Visible warts on cervix, labia, or penis or around anus
  - Visual identification, may have no symptoms
- Cervical infection associated with increased risk of cervical cancer; head, neck, and rectal cancers associated with other sites of infection

Gonorrhea
- > 350,000 new cases reported to CDC in 2006
  - Estimates of true infection rate is twice that number
- Caused by the bacteria *Neisseria gonorrhoeae*
- Painful urination
- Purulent vaginal or penile discharge

Syphilis
- 36,000 reported cases in United States in 2006
- Caused by the bacteria *Treponema pallidum*
- Primary stage
  - Painless sore = chancre
    - Heals without treatment in 3–6 weeks but infection persists if not treated
- Secondary stage
  - Nonitchy rash, classically on palms and soles
  - May have fever, swollen lymph glands, weight loss, fatigue, headaches
  - Rash and symptoms will disappear but infection persists if not treated = latent stage
- Late stage
  - Damage to brain, internal organs, blood vessels, bones
  - May cause death

Demographics
- Adolescents with high rates and high risks of STIs
- 50% of STIs in < 25-year-olds
- Females 15–19 years have highest rates of gonorrhea and chlamydia

Risk Factors
- Unprotected sexual contact with infected individual
- Young adolescents (< 15 years)
  - Increased predisposition to infection, increased rates of unprotected sexual activity, unlikely to seek health care
- Male homosexuals
- Those injecting drugs

Prevention and Screening
- Education and counseling about avoidance by changing sexual behaviors
- Identification of asymptomatic patients or those unlikely to seek care
- Prevention via pre-exposure immunization
  - Human papilloma virus
  - Hepatitis A and B

Assessment

- Diagnosis of infected individuals
  - Microscopic evaluation of vaginal or penile drainage
  - Swabs of penis or cervix

Management

- Treatment: Single-dose treatment at time of diagnosis most efficacious
  - Gonorrhea
    - Single IM dose of ceftriaxone
    - Assume *Chlamydia* infection and treat
  - *Chlamydia*
    - Single dose of azithromycin orally
  - Syphilis
    - Single dose of IM penicillin
    - Alternative medications available if allergic for all of above
  - Genital herpes
    - No curative therapies
    - Suppressive therapies for repeated outbreaks
      · Does not cure or limit risk of spread
  - Human papilloma virus
    - No treatment currently recommended
    - Virus typically taken care of by body and goes away on own
- Disease control
  - Evaluation, treatment, and counseling for sex partners of those with sexually transmitted infections
- Mandatory reporting to local health department
  - Consult your state's guidelines
  - Syphilis, gonorrhea, chlamydia, HIV infection, and AIDS are currently reportable in all states

Outcomes and Follow-Up

- Excellent outcome if early identification and curative therapy available
- Pelvic inflammatory disease and epididymitis as complications of untreated STIs
  - Can lead to infertility or sterility
- As above, education re: mode of transmission, safe sex practices, identification and treatment of at-risk partners
- Careful screening for cervical cancer for those with history of HPV infection

REFERENCES

American Academy of Pediatrics, Committee on Quality Improvement, Subcommittee on Urinary Tract Infection. (1999). *Practice parameter: The diagnosis, treatment and evaluation of the initial urinary tract infection in febrile infants and young children.* Retrieved from http://aappolicy. aappublications.org/cgi/reprint/pediatrics;103/4/843.pdf

Centers for Disease Control and Prevention. (2008). *Sexually transmitted diseases.* Retrieved from http://www.cdc.gov/std/default.htm

Kliegman, R.M., Behrman, R. E., Jenson, H. B., & Stanton, B. F. (Eds.) (2007). *Nelson's textbook of pediatrics* (18th ed.). Philadelphia: Saunders Elsevier.

National Institutes of Health: National Kidney and Urologic Diseases Information Clearinghouse. (2008). *Childhood nephrotic syndrome* (NIH Publication No. 08–4695). Retrieved from http:// kidney.niddk.nih.gov/kudiseases/pubs/childkidneydiseases/nephrotic_syndrom/

Potts, N. L., & Mandleco, B. L. (Eds.). (2007). *Pediatric nursing: Caring for children and their families* (2nd ed.). Clifton Park, NY: Tomson.

13

Endocrine Disorders

Karen Corlett, MSN, RN-BC, CPNP-AC/PC, PNP-BC

DIABETES MELLITUS

Description
- Elevated blood glucose levels related to lack of or insensitivity to insulin produced by the body
- Classified as Type 1 or Type 2 diabetes
  - Type 1 diabetes
    - Inadequate insulin production by the pancreas
    - Requires insulin replacement therapy
  - Type 2 diabetes
    - Cells insensitive to effects of insulin = insulin resistance
    - Pancreas eventually fails due to need for high insulin production
    - May eventually require insulin replacement therapy

Etiology
- Inadequate insulin production by the pancreas
  - Typically autoimmune destruction of the beta cells of the pancreas
- Altered action of insulin
- Combination of both of the above

Incidence and Demographics
- 1 in 400–600 children/adolescents have Type 1 diabetes in the United States
- 0.2% or > 175,000 people < 20 years of age in the United States have diabetes
- CDC estimated that 20.6 million, or 9.6% of the U.S. population > 20 years old, had diabetes in 2005
  - Increasing frequency of diagnosis in children and adolescents
- Type 1 diabetes: 5%–10% of all diagnosed diabetes
- Type 2 diabetes: 90%–95% of all diagnosed diabetes

Risk Factors
Type 1 Diabetes
- Younger age at onset
- Autoimmune, genetic, and environmental components not well defined

Type 2 Diabetes
- Older age
- Obesity, lack of physical activity
  - Asian populations develop Type 2 diabetes at lower body weights than other groups
- Positive family history, history of gestational diabetes
- Race/ethnicity
  - Pacific Islanders, Native Americans, Blacks, Asian Americans, Latino/Hispanic Americans are all high-risk groups

Prevention and Screening
Type 2 diabetes preventable through diet and exercise

Assessment
Type 1 Diabetes Presentation
- Excessive thirst and urination (polyuria and polydipsia)
  - Elevated serum glucose levels exceed renal threshold
  - Glucosuria develops
    - Osmotic diuresis from glucosuria
  - Increased urine water losses → increased thirst
- Dehydration
- Increased food intake and weight loss (polyphagia)
- Abdominal pain, vomiting
- Significantly elevated serum glucose

Type 2 Diabetes Presentation
- Two elevated fasting glucose levels > 125 mg/dL
- Two elevated random glucose levels > 200 mg/dL
- Acanthosis nigricans
  - Soft hyperpigmented patches of skin
  - Classically back of neck, axillae

Diabetic Ketoacidosis
- May be presenting event or complication of diabetes
- Severe hyperglycemia due to lack of insulin
- Dehydration
- Acidosis
- Coma if not recognized or treated early enough
- Kussmaul respirations
    - Deep, rapid respirations
    - Acetone breath

Hypoglycemia
- Low serum glucose
- Inadequate food intake and/or
- Excessive exercise and/or
- Too much insulin
- Treat with fast-acting carbohydrate to raise serum glucose quickly
    - Plus complex carbohydrate to prevent rebound hypoglycemia

Management
Type 1 Diabetes
- Insulin replacement
    - Multiple daily injections or continuous infusion via pump
- Dietary modifications
- Goal is control of serum glucose
    - Home glucose monitoring several times/day
    - Glycosylated hemoglobin (HgbA1c)
        · Measures glucose control over previous 2–3 months

Education of Patient and Family
- Disease process
- Insulin action
    - Insulin delivery method
- Interaction of insulin and food
- Effect of exercise on food and insulin needs
- Home blood glucose monitoring and targeted goals
- Signs and symptoms of hypoglycemia and hyperglycemia
    - Signs and symptoms of diabetic ketoacidosis
- Importance of having fast-acting carbohydrate available at all times
- Psychosocial support
    - Counselors
    - Diabetes camps

Type 2 Diabetes
- Weight loss
- Dietary modifications
- Regular exercise
- Oral antihyperglycemic agents if not controlled with diet and exercise
- Subcutaneous insulin delivery if not controlled with above
- Patient and family education

Avoidance of Complications
- Team approach
- Patient, family, and care providers as partners in care
  - Pediatrician, endocrinologist, certified diabetes educator, nutritionist
- Tight glucose control
  - Maintenance of targeted HgbA1c

Outcomes and Follow-Up
- Home blood glucose monitoring reviews
  - HgbA1c monitoring 2–4 times/year
  - Each 1% drop in HgbA1c can decrease risk of microvascular complications by as much as 40%
- Routine clinic appointments
- Avoidance of, and monitoring for, complications:
  - Retinopathy and blindness
  - Heart disease and stroke
  - Hypertension
  - Kidney disease
  - Neuropathy
  - Poor wound healing, skin ulcers, amputations
  - Gum disease
  - Pregnancy and newborn infant complications

GROWTH DISORDERS

Causing delayed or abnormal physical growth patterns

Description
A variety of disorders causing abnormal somatic growth

Etiology
Causes can be genetic or environmental

Prevention and Screening
No prevention or screening indicated

Assessment
Bone and Cartilage Dysplasias: Disproportionate Growth Disorders
ACHONDROPLASIA
- 1:26,000 births, autosomal dominant transmission
- Very short stature, large head, flat midface, short proximal limbs, small thorax, multiple vertebral and joint anomalies

HYPOCHONDROPLASIA
- Less marked short stature
- Cranial, vertebral, joint, and limb anomalies
- Growth until age 2 years may be near normal

Secondary Growth Disorders
MALNUTRITION
- Lack of nutrients lead to poor growth
- Chronic or intermittent condition
- Significant intercurrent illness with disruption of adequate caloric intake
- Interruptions during critical periods of growth may permanently impact growth

Growth Hormone Deficiency
- Congenital or acquired (after central nervous system [CNS] tumor/resection/radiation)
- Slow somatic growth and maturation
- Bone age delayed for chronological age
- Diagnosed by elaborate stimulation test with frequent lab draws

Constitutional Growth Delay
- Slow growth
- Normal pattern of growth but delayed in reaching age-appropriate goals
  - Growth curve maintained
- Late puberty
- Achieve typical adult height

Familial Short Stature
- Remains at about 5th percentile for age throughout childhood
- Normal bone age for chronological age
- Typical age when puberty occurs
- Short adult height but on target for his or her genetic potential

Genetic Disorders Associated With Short Stature
TURNER SYNDROME
- Girls with 45x chromosomal makeup
- Short adult stature
- Short webbed neck, low hairline, flat midface, small jaw, prominent ears, widely spaced nipples, lymphedema of hands and feet, coarctation of the aorta
- No secondary sex characteristics without hormone therapy
  - Ovarian failure
- Normal intelligence

PRADER-WILLI SYNDROME
- Abnormality on chromosome 15
- Small for gestational age and poor growth until age 2 years
- Age 2 or older, weight gain outpaces rate of height gain
  - Obesity develops
- Short adult stature
- Developmental delay

DOWN SYNDROME
- Three 21st chromosomes
- 1 in 600 live births
- Simian creases of hands, short digits, large tongue, low-set ears, epicanthal folds, cardiac disease, congenital genitourinary disorders, developmental delay, hypotonia
- Slightly smaller birth weights and lengths
- Slower but steady growth throughout childhood
- Achieve shorter than average adult height
- Thyroid dysfunction frequent
- Varying degrees of developmental delay

NOONAN SYNDROME
- Autosomal dominant, abnormality of chromosome 12
- Webbed neck, low posterior hairline, ear malformations, pulmonary stenosis, hematologic disorders
- Small male genitalia with undescended testicles
- Delayed puberty
- Mental retardation in ~30%, speech and language delay, delayed motor skills
- Short adult height

Overgrowth Syndromes
BECKWITH-WIEDEMANN SYNDROME
- Abnormality of chromosome 11
- Large for gestational age
- Large tongue, large organs, nevus on face, ear abnormalities, small midface, umbilical hernias
- Hypoglycemia
  - Close neonatal serum blood glucose monitoring

SOTOS SYNDROME (CEREBRAL GIGANTISM)
- Large for gestational age
- Developmental delay, macrocephaly, prominent ears, large jaw and chin, high palate, thick subcutaneous tissues, large hands and feet
- Stay above 97th percentile for height on growth chart
- Advanced bone age, early puberty
  - Overgrowth is stopped early, often normal adult height

GROWTH HORMONE EXCESS
- Concern for growth hormone-secreting pituitary tumor
- Increased height if before growth plates close, coarse features and thick bones if after growth plates fuse

KLINEFELTER SYNDROME
- Two or more X chromosomes in males (47 XXY most common)
- 1 in 500–1,000 live births
- Tall stature as adolescents
- Long limbs, mental retardation, behavior difficulties
- Low testosterone secretion from underdeveloped testes
    - Small genitalia, delayed puberty, infertility

MARFAN SYNDROME
- Autosomal dominant inheritance pattern
    - Locus on chromosome 15
- Collagen disorder
- Joint laxity, scoliosis, lens and retinal detachments, aortic disorders, long fingers and toes, pectus deformities
- Tall with long arms and legs
- Decreased life span due to cardiac/aortic abnormalities

Management
Meticulous Records of Height and Weight
- Appropriate growth charts for age and condition
- Length until age 2, then standing height
- Follow percentile growth
    - Weight for height
- Body mass index
    - BMI
    - Plot on BMI growth charts

Evaluate for Cause of Growth Abnormalities
- Somatic causes as above
- Nutritional deficits or excesses
- Environmental or economic influences

Referrals as Appropriate
- Geneticist
- Endocrinologist
    - Growth hormone therapy in appropriate patients
        - Daily injections of human growth hormone
- Nutritionist
- Pediatric weight management or healthy lifestyle programs
    - Education and support
    - Involve entire family

Outcomes and Follow-Up
- Goal is for child to reach average adult height whenever possible
- Continue meticulous monitoring of height and weight
- Management of associated comorbidities
  - Encourage specialty care referral and follow-up

GROWTH DISORDERS

Causing alterations in maturation.

Description
Abnormalities in growth causing premature or delayed puberty

Etiology
Genetic, familial, environmental, and/or hormonal influences

Incidence and Demographics
Precocious puberty occurs in 4%–5% of children

Risk Factors
Inadequate or excess secretion of, or sensitivity to, the sex hormones

Prevention and Screening
- No prevention or screening indicated

Assessment
Precocious Puberty
- Development of secondary sexual characteristics in girls before age 6–7
- Development of secondary sexual characteristics in boys before age 10

Delayed Puberty
- No breast tissue in girls by age 13
- No testicular enlargement in boys by age 14
- > 5 years from onset until completion of puberty
  - Completion is menarche in girls
  - Completion of genital development in boys

May Be Normal Variant
- Referral to pediatric endocrinologist
- Evaluation of bone age
- Evaluation of gonadal, pituitary, and adrenal function

Management

Precocious Puberty
- Gonadotropin-releasing hormone therapy
    - To turn off current pituitary excess
    - Monthly depot injections most common modality

Delayed Puberty
- Testosterone replacement by injection in boys
- Cyclical replacement with estrogen and progesterone in girls

Education and Psychosocial Support
- Diagnosis
- Causation
- Treatment modalities
- Physical differences

Outcomes and Follow-Up
- Goals of therapy:
    - Optimum growth in precocious puberty
    - Optimum pubertal development in delayed puberty
    - Identification and management of any uncovered diseases/syndromes

DIABETES INSIPIDUS

Description
- Antidiuretic hormone (ADH) deficiency
- Large amounts of urine output
    - ADH not present to cause reabsorption of water from the collecting tubules in the kidney
- Presentation
    - Polyuria, polydipsia
    - Dehydration if unable to keep up with fluid losses
    - Electrolyte abnormalities due to fluid losses and urinary losses of electrolytes

Etiology
- Pituitary tumors or their removal
- Head trauma or brain injury
- Hypothalamic or pituitary disorders

Incidence and Demographics
- Unknown

Risk Factors
- CNS malformations or anomalies
- Head injury or trauma
- Neurosurgical procedures near the pituitary gland

Prevention and Screening
- No prevention or screening indicated

Assessment
- Symptoms of polyuria and polydipsia
  - Preference for water
  - Bedwetting, especially if after a period of nighttime dryness
- Evaluation for signs and symptoms of dehydration
- Urine studies find dilute urine
  - Low specific gravity
  - Low urine osmolality
- Serum electrolyte evaluation
  - Excess losses with large volume of urine output
  - Serum concentration due to excess water losses
    - Hypernatremia most serious threat
    - At risk for seizures
- Close monitoring during any diagnostic tests
  - Water deprivation test
    - Evaluation of serum ADH levels
  - Close monitoring of intake vs. output, weight, electrolytes

Management
- Allow older child free access to fluids
  - Can be well-controlled without medication if normal thirst mechanism and ability to get to fluids
  - Frequent urination can be disruptive to normal activities
- ADH supplementation
  - Nasal inhalation of ADH for long-term management
    - Clear nasal passage before administration
    - Inhale with administration
    - Lie on dosed side for several minutes postadministration
    - Enteral and IV routes available
  - Long-acting drug
    - Polyuria will recur in several hours once drug effect subsides
    - Documentation helps determine dosing interval
  - Goals of therapy
    - Control of polyuria
      - Nighttime dryness for preschoolers and older children
    - Acceptable electrolyte balance
    - Careful monitoring as treatment is initiated/adjusted
  - Close monitoring if gastrointestinal illnesses or periods when unable to drink

PITUITARY DISORDERS

Description
- Lack of or excess secretion of pituitary hormones
- Anterior pituitary hormones
  - Thyroid-stimulating hormone
  - Growth hormone
  - Adrenocorticotropic hormone (ACTH)
  - Gonadotropins
  - Follicle-stimulating hormone
    Luteinizing hormone
  - Prolactin
  - Melanocyte-stimulating hormone
- Posterior pituitary hormones
  - Antidiuretic hormone
  - Oxytocin

Etiology
- Congenital pituitary disorder
- Head trauma or surgical injury

Incidence and Demographics
- Rare but difficult to determine specific incidences

Risk Factors
- Brain tumors or resections of tumors
- Traumatic brain injury

Prevention and Screening
- No prevention or screening indicated

Assessment
- Hypopituitarism
  - Lack of somatic growth
  - Delayed puberty
- Hyperpituitarism
  - Excessive growth
    - Height if before growth plates close
    - Large and thick bones of mandible, joints, feet, if after growth plate closure
- Serum hormone levels
- Radiologic evaluation of bone age
- Careful monitoring and plotting of growth parameters

Management
- Referral to pediatric endocrine specialist
  - Evaluate cause of hypo- or hyperpituitarism
- Hormone replacement therapies as ordered

- Growth hormone most common replacement therapy
  - Daily subcutaneous injections
  - Education of patient and family re: risks/benefits
  - Education of patient and family re: administration techniques
  - Facilitate reimbursement of costs of therapy
    - Insurance approval
    - Adjunct programs to help defray costs

Outcomes and Follow-Up
- Goal is normal serum hormone levels or normal effects of missing or low level hormones
- Follow serum hormone levels
- Follow height and weight closely

THYROID DISORDERS

Description
Abnormal serum thyroid levels

Etiology
- Congenital or acquired hypothyroidism
- Abnormal stimulation from pituitary gland
  - Pituitary tumors
- Autoimmune attack on thyroid gland

Incidence and Demographics
- Congenital hypothyroidism in ~1:4,000 live births
- Graves disease in childhood most common in 5–16 year olds
  - Girls > boys

Risk Factors
- Not well-defined

Assessment
Congenital Hypothyroidism
- Abnormal newborn screen results
  - Low T3 and free T4
- Many infants are asymptomatic
- Associated symptoms:
  - Large, thick tongue; large anterior fontanelle; umbilical hernia; constipation; prolonged hyperbilirubinemia; hypotonia; dry and scaly skin; hypothermia
- Start therapy urgently to avoid further brain damage

Hypothyroidism in Older Children
SYMPTOMS
- Poor growth, or weight gain if grown
- Constipation
- Dry, scaly skin

- Hypothermia, sense of always being cold
- Thin hair
- Fatigue
- Hypotonia
- Delayed puberty
- Enlarged thyroid (goiter) in some
- Low T3 and T4
- Low or normal thyroid-stimulating hormone (TSH) depending on cause

Hyperthyroidism
- Graves disease most common
  - Autoimmune disease
  - Antibodies to thyroid gland mimic TSH and cause excessive stimulation and release of thyroid hormone
- Symptoms:
  - Goiter
  - Increased growth, or weight loss if grown
  - Advanced bone age
  - Tachycardia
  - Insomnia, hyperactivity
  - Emotional lability
  - Exophthalmus and proptosis
- Characterized by exacerbations and remissions

Management
Hypothyroidism
- Thyroid supplementation with l-thyroxine
- Reevaluation of serum blood levels
  - Aggressive treatment and monitoring in infants to avoid further brain damage
- No commercially available liquid preparations
  - Crush pill and dissolve dose in liquid
  - Parent education re dosing
  - Avoid giving with soy formulas—decreases absorption
- Careful monitoring of growth parameters

Hyperthyroidism
- Treatment options
  - Antithyroid medications (propylthiouracil [PTU])
  - Radioactive iodine therapy
  - Subtotal thyroidectomy
- None without risks
  - Facilitate family education re: risks and benefits of proposed therapies
- Continued monitoring of thyroid levels even after therapy complete
  - May have residual hyperthyroidism
  - May have iatrogenic hypothyroidism
- Continued monitoring of growth parameters
- Evaluation for additional autoimmune disorders

Outcomes and Follow-Up
- Goal is normalization of serum hormone levels through treatment or supplemental medication
  - Frequent follow up and evaluation of serum levels
- Resumption of normal growth pattern

REFERENCES

American Diabetes Association. (2008). Diagnosis and classification of diabetes mellitus. *Diabetes Care, 31*, S55–S60.

Centers for Disease Control and Prevention. (2005). *National diabetes fact sheet: General information and national estimates on diabetes in the U.S., 2005.* Atlanta, GA: U.S. Government Printing Office.

Herman-Giddens, M. E., Slora, E. J., Wasserman, R. C., Bourdony, M. V., Koch, G. G., & Hasemeier, C. M. (1997). Secondary sexual characteristics and menses in young girls seen in office practice: A study from the Pediatric Research in Office Settings Network. *Pediatrics, 99*(4), 505–512.

Kappy, M. S., Allen, D. B., & Geffner, M. E. (Eds.). (2005). *Principles and practice of pediatric endocrinology.* Springfield, IL: Charles C. Thomas.

Peterson, K., Silverstein, J., Kaufman, F., & Warren-Boulton, E. (2007). Management of type 2 diabetes in youth: An update. *American Family Physician, 76*, 658–666.

Potts, N. L., & Mandleco, B. L. (Eds.). (2007). *Pediatric nursing: Caring for children and their families* (2nd ed.). Clifton Park, NY: Tomson.

14

Hematologic Disorders

Clara J. Richardson, MSN, RN-BC

SEPSIS

Description
Sepsis, also called occult bacteremia, is defined as the presence of a microorganism in the bloodstream.

Etiology
The most common causes of sepsis in children are *Haemophilus influenzae* type b and *Streptococcus pneumoniae*.

Incidence and Demographics
The incidence of sepsis has greatly decreased since the development of vaccines against these causative organisms, but remains at 1.6%–1.8% in children younger than 36 months of age. Sepsis is more prevalent in infants younger than 90 days and most prevalent in those younger than 29 days.

Risk Factors
- Infection
- Maternal fever at the time of delivery
- Maternal history of group B streptococcal infection or herpes simplex virus infection during pregnancy
- Incomplete immunizations

Prevention and Screening
Sepsis may be prevented by treatment of maternal infections during pregnancy and adherence to immunization schedule; no screening indicated.

Assessment
History
- History of risk factors
- Presence of physical symptoms
- Age

Physical Exam
- Fever
- Hypothermia in neonates
- Apnea in neonates
- Cyanosis
- Hyper- or hypoventilation
- Decreased activity
- Lethargy
- Irritability progressing to lethargy
- Poor muscle tone
- Decreased perfusion
- Tachycardia
- Subtle changes described as "not looking or acting right"

Diagnostic Studies
- White blood cell count shows elevation, increased band cells, elevated absolute neutrophil count (ANA)
- Blood culture to identify microorganism
- Culture of any areas with bodily discharge
- Urinalysis and culture may reveal urinary origin of infection
- Lumbar puncture may reveal central nervous system infection
- Chest radiography to rule out pneumonia

Management
Invasive
- No invasive management indicated

Nonpharmacologic
- Light clothing
- Cool cloth for fever
- Extra oral fluids

Pharmacologic
- Two broad-spectrum antibiotic to cover gram positive and gram negative organisms, such as Ceftriaxone (Rocephin) and Cefotaxime (Claforan)
- Acetaminophen or ibuprofen for fever
- Intravenous therapy to maintain fluid and electrolyte balance

Patient/Family Education
- Disease process and treatment plan
- Medication administration
- Care of child with fever
- Strategies to prevent spread of infection
- Recommended immunization schedule

Outcomes and Follow-Up
- The child will receive prompt treatment and recover fully.
- The child will maintain fluid and electrolyte balance.
- The child's temperature will return to normal.
- The family will verbalize understanding of disease process and treatment plan.
- The family will demonstrate effective medication administration and fever care.
- The family will identify strategies to prevent spread of infection.
- The family will demonstrate compliance with recommended immunization schedule.

IRON DEFICIENCY ANEMIA

Description
Iron deficiency anemia (IDA) is decreased number of red blood cells and/or reduced hemoglobin concentration due to inadequate supply, loss, or impaired absorption of iron.

Etiology
The main cause of iron deficiency anemia in children is nutritional deficit of iron. Iron is transferred from the mother to the fetus during the last trimester of gestation. These stores are adequate for the first 5–6 months in full-term infants. When iron stores are depleted, the production of hemoglobin is decreased, as is the oxygen-carrying capacity of the blood.

Incidence and Demographics
Iron deficiency anemia affects 7% of children age 1–2 years, 5% of children age 3–5 years, 4% of children age 6–11 years. Long-term effects of IDA in children may include visual, hearing, and cognitive impairment.

Risk Factors
- Prematurity or low birth weight
- High intake of unfortified cow's milk
- Immigrants from developing countries
- Low socioeconomic level
- Black, Native American, Alaskan Native

Prevention and Screening

- Routine iron supplementation for infants age 6–12 months who have identified risk factors
- Prenatal vitamins for all pregnant women
- Breastfeeding
- Iron-fortified formula
- Iron-enriched foods

Screening

- U.S. Preventive Services Task Force (USPSTF) recommends screening of symptomatic children
- Centers for Disease Control and Prevention (CDC) recommends screening of children with risk factors
- American Academy of Pediatrics (AAP) recommends screening of all infants 9–12 months of age and again 6 months later, children with risk factors, and annually for children 2–5 years of age

Assessment

History

- Specific nutritional history reveals inadequate iron intake
- Presence of risk factors
- Frequent infections

Physical Exam

- Pallor
- Glossitis, inflammation of the tongue
- Elevated pulse and respiratory rates
- Heart murmur
- Enlarged liver or spleen

Diagnostic Studies

- Hemoglobin <11 g/dL in children 6 months–4.9 years and <11.5 g/dL in children 5–11.9 years
- Decreased mean corpuscular volume (MCV)
- Elevated red cell distribution width (RDW)
- Decreased reticulocyte count
- Decreased serum ferritin, serum iron, or transferrin levels
- Elevated total iron-binding capacity (TIBC)
- Elevated free erythrocyte protoporphyrin (FEP)

Management

Invasive

- No invasive management indicated

Nonpharmacologic

- Iron-fortified diet
- No cow's milk before 12 months of age
- Limit milk intake in toddlers to 2–3 cups per day

Pharmacologic
- Oral iron supplement (Fer-In-Sol)

Patient/Family Education
- Disorder and treatment plan
- Safe administration of iron supplement
  - Liquid forms may stain teeth and should be given far back in mouth with teeth brushed afterwards
  - Citrus fruit or juice will enhance absorption
  - Tea or antacids will decrease absorption
  - Stools will be dark green or black
- Diet recommendations

Outcomes and Follow-Up
- The child's lab tests will return to normal.
- The child's intake of iron-rich foods will increase.
- The child's intake will reflect recommended dietary allowances.
- The family will verbalize understanding of disorder and treatment plan.
- The family will demonstrate effective medication administration.

SICKLE CELL ANEMIA

Description
Sickle cell anemia is the homozygous form of sickle cell disease (SCD), an autosomal recessive inherited blood disorder.

Etiology
Children with sickle cell disease produce hemoglobin S in addition to normal adult hemoglobin A. A structural defect in the ß-globin chain of the hemoglobin S molecule causes the red blood cells to become sickle-shaped when exposed to a state of decreased oxygen. These stiff, curved cells can obstruct the small vessels, causing tissue ischemia and organ damage. Vaso-occlusion involves a complex interaction of sickled cells, platelets, leukocytes, plasma components, and vascular endothelium.

Sickle cell anemia is characterized by acute episodes called crises. The most common is a vaso-occlusive crisis with an area of obstruction and ischemia. In a sequestration crisis, large amounts of blood pool in the spleen or liver causing shock. An aplastic crisis, a severe anemia, occurs when there is a decrease in red blood cell production usually triggered by an infection. If sickled cells obstruct a major blood vessel in the brain, the child experiences a cerebrovascular accident, or stroke. Repeat episodes of acute chest syndrome, the result of obstruction of the small vessels in the lungs, can cause restrictive lung disease and pulmonary hypertension.

Incidence and Demographics
Sickle cell disease affects 1 in 375 Blacks and 1 in 36,000 Hispanic newborns. Sequestration crisis is most prevalent between the ages of 2 months and 5 years. The average life span of an individual with sickle cell anemia has increased to 50 years. 11% of children with sickle cell anemia will have a stroke, most commonly between the ages of 2 and 10 years.

Risk Factors

Sickling may result when the child experiences infection, fever, dehydration, acidosis, hypoxia, stress, or cold.

Prevention and Screening

- Prevention of infection and other risk factors
- Screening of newborns
    - Thin-layer isoelectric focusing (IEF)
    - High-performance liquid chromatography (HPLC)
- Screening of children with transcranial Doppler ultrasound to identify stroke risk
    - Starting at age 2 years
    - Children with transcranial blood-flow velocity (TBV) equal to or greater than 200 cm per second are considered at high risk
- Retinal screening beginning at age 10 years
- Screening with transthoracic Doppler echocardiography for pulmonary hypertension in older adolescents and adults
- Screening for carrier state of parents and sexual partners of diagnosed individuals accompanied by genetic counseling

Assessment

History

- Paleness
- Fatigue
- Growth delay

Physical Exam

VASO-OCCLUSIVE CRISIS

- Severe pain
- Hematuria
- Priapism (painful penile erection)
- Dactylitis (painful swelling of hands and feet) in children < 2 years of age

SEQUESTRATION CRISIS

- Hepatomegaly
- Splenomegaly
- Circulatory collapse

APLASTIC CRISIS

- Pallor
- Fatigue and muscle weakness
- Shortness of breath
- Systolic heart murmur

CEREBROVASCULAR ACCIDENT (STROKE)
- Behavioral changes
- Prolonged headache
- Sudden weakness or numbness
- Vision or speech loss
- Dizziness or falls

PULMONARY HYPERTENSION
- Dyspnea
- Hypoxemia
- Increased intensity of second heart sound

ACUTE CHEST SYNDROME
- Chest pain
- Fever
- Wheezing
- Dyspnea or tachypnea
- Cough

Diagnostic Studies
- Chest radiography
- Blood and sputum cultures
- Complete blood counts and serum chemistry
- Hemoglobin S concentration with Hgb electrophoresis pre- and posttransfusion therapy
- Annual evaluation of renal, liver, and pulmonary function

Management
Invasive
- Hematopoietic cell transplant is curative for sickle cell disease, but not widely used due to lack of identical donors and associated toxicity of current treatment protocols

Nonpharmacologic
- Oxygen only when hypoxia present
- Incentive spirometry while awake
- Monitor oxygen saturation
- Warm compresses for painful areas
- Bedrest and passive range of motion during pain crisis
- Adequate oral fluid intake

Pharmacologic
- Prophylactic antibiotics to prevent infection in children 2 months to 5 years of age
  - Oral penicillin V potassium (Veetids) daily
  - IM penicillin G benzathine (Bicillin L-A) every 3 weeks can be substituted
  - Administration continued past 5 years if child has history of invasive pneumococcal infection or splenectomy

- Immunization to prevent pneumococcal infections
  - 7-valent pneumococcal conjugate vaccine (PCV, Prevnar) for children under 2 years of age
  - 23-valent polysaccharide pneumococcal vaccine (PPV) if 2 years or older
  - Revaccination 3–5 years later
- Annual influenza immunization for children 6 months and older
- Meningococcal vaccination for children 2 years and older
- Pain management
  - For mild to moderate pain: Acetaminophen or ibuprofen
  - For more severe pain: Codeine, morphine, hydromorphone (Dilaudid), oxycodone
  - Avoid meperidine (Demerol), a central nervous system stimulant, because children with sickle cell disease are more likely to have seizures
- Hydroxyurea for older adolescents who have three or more moderate to severe vaso-occlusive painful episodes per year
  - To increase levels of hemoglobin F, which does not sickle
  - To decrease adhesion of red cells
- Intravenous therapy to maintain fluid and electrolyte balance and to decrease capillary obstruction
- Broad-spectrum antibiotics for infection
- Bronchodilators for restrictive airway disease
- Blood transfusion therapy
  - Episodic transfusions for acute chest syndrome, multi-organ failure, splenic or hepatic sequestration, aplastic crisis, major surgical procedures, stroke, symptomatic anemia, complications of pregnancy
  - Chronic transfusions for children at high risk for stroke, prevention of stroke recurrence, chronic heart failure, pulmonary hypertension, prevention of recurrent splenic sequestration
- Chelation therapy for iron overload resulting from chronic blood transfusion therapy

Patient/Family Education
- Disease process and treatment plan
- Genetic implications
- Signs of crisis, stroke, pulmonary hypertension, acute chest syndrome
- Signs of infection and prevention strategies
- Signs of dehydration and prevention strategies
- Medication administration
- Immunization protocol
- Screening protocols for stroke, retinal damage, pulmonary hypertension

Outcomes and Follow-Up
- The child will experience prompt treatment for infection or crisis.
- The child will experience prompt treatment for stroke, acute chest syndrome, pulmonary hypertension.
- The child will experience effective pain management of acute and chronic pain
- The child will maintain hydration.
- The child will demonstrate balanced rest and activity.

- The family will verbalize understanding of disease process and treatment plan.
- The family will verbalize understanding of the genetic implications of sickle cell disease.
- The family will identify signs of crisis, infection, dehydration.
- The family will demonstrate strategies to prevent infection and dehydration.
- The family will demonstrate medication administration.
- The family will demonstrate compliance with immunization and screening protocols.

IDIOPATHIC THROMBOCYTOPENIC PURPURA

Description
Idiopathic thrombocytopenic purpura (ITP) is an autoimmune disorder resulting in thrombocytopenia, low platelet count. By definition, acute ITP lasts less than 6 months and the chronic form lasts longer than 6 months.

Etiology
The exact etiology of ITP is unknown. The B-cells produce antiplatelet antibodies, which destroy platelets.

Incidence and Demographics
The incidence of acute ITP is approximately 2.5–5 per 100,000 children each year, with the peak incidence at 5.5 years of age. Acute ITP is most common between the ages of 1 and 10 years, while chronic ITP more commonly occurs in children older than 9 years. About half of the children who have acute ITP between the ages of 10 and 18 years will develop the chronic form. The disease is more prevalent in the spring and early summer.

Risk Factors
No identified risk factors

Prevention and Screening
No prevention or screening

Assessment
History
- Prior viral illness
- Sudden onset of bruising, petechiae, nose bleeds

Physical Exam
- Bruising and petechiae
- Hemorrhagic blisters in the mouth called wet purpura

Diagnostic Studies
- Low platelet count

Management
Invasive
- Splenectomy for life-threatening bleeding or in chronic ITP

Nonpharmacologic
- Avoid contact sports and activities likely to result in falls
- Avoid aspirin and ibuprofen
- Platelet infusions for life-threatening bleeding
- Packed red blood cell transfusion for decreased hemoglobin with significant bleeding

Pharmacologic
CORTICOSTEROIDS
- Prednisone
- Methylprednisolone (Solu-Medrol)

INTRAVENOUS IMMUNE GLOBULIN (IG) TO INCREASE NUMBER OF PLATELETS
- Rh(D) immune globulin (WinRho) only in Rh-positive children
- Monoclonal antibiodies in cases that do not respond to other treatment

Patient/Family Education
- Disease process and treatment plan
- Strategies to prevent bleeding
- Medication administration

Outcomes and Follow-Up
- The child will not experience bleeding episode.
- The child's platelet level will increase.
- The family will verbalize understanding of the disease process and treatment plan.
- The family will utilize strategies to prevent bleeding.
- The family will demonstrate effective medication administration.

HEMOPHILIA

Description
Hemophilia is a group of X-linked recessive bleeding disorders. The most common forms are hemophilia A—factor VIII deficiency, and hemophilia B—factor IX deficiency.

Etiology
Both factors are necessary for blood coagulation. Factor VIII is produced in the liver and is required for the formation of thromboplastin. Children with hemophilia bleed for longer periods, not more profusely.

Incidence and Demographics
The incidence of hemophilia A is 1 in 5,000 live male births; hemophilia B occurs in 1 in 30,000 live male births. Hemophilia A is classified by the level of factor VIII activity (see Table 14–1).

Table 14-1. Hemophilia Classification by Factor VIII Activity

Classification	Factor VIII Activity	Prevalence
Mild	5%–40%	31%
Moderate	1%–5%	26%
Severe	<1%	43%

The life expectancy of the individual with hemophilia has increased from 30 years in the 1980s to about 65 years of age. The most serious complication of hemophilia is the development of inhibitor antibodies against factor VIII, which happens in about 6% of those with the disorder.

Risk Factors
Maternal carrier status

Prevention and Screening
There is no prevention, but genetic screening for the disease and carrier status is possible.

Assessment
History
• Excessive bleeding with circumcision

MILD HEMOPHILIA
  • Hemorrhage after major trauma
  • Hemorrhage after surgery

MODERATE HEMOPHILIA
  • Infrequent spontaneous bleeding
  • Bleeding after mild trauma

SEVERE HEMOPHILIA
  • Spontaneous bleeding resulting in hemarthrosis, soft tissue hematoma, intracranial hemorrhage
  • Frequent nose bleeds and bruising

Physical Exam
• Hemarthrosis: Bleeding into the joint
  – Most common and severe manifestation
  – Repeat joint bleeds result in permanent deformity
  – Joint stiffness, tingling, ache, decreased mobility
  – Joint warmth, redness, swelling, severe pain
• Bleeding into mouth, neck, chest may lead to airway obstruction
• Intracranial hemorrhage
  – Headache
  – Slurred speech
  – Loss of consciousness

- Bleeding in the gastrointestinal tract
  - Black, tarry stools
  - Anemia
- Hematomas of the spine may result in paralysis
- Hematuria

Diagnostic Studies
- Factor activity assays during fetal period or from umbilical cord blood at delivery for children of carrier parents
- Coagulation factor assays to identify specific factor deficiency
- Prolonged partial thromboplastin time (PTT)
- Screening for HIV and hepatitis for those receiving factor replacement before 1989

Management
Invasive
- No invasive management indicated

Nonpharmacologic
- RICE: Rest, ice, compression, elevation
- Avoid passive range of motion during acute episode
- Avoid aspirin, ibuprofen, heparin, and warfarin (Coumadin)
- Prevention of injury in toddlers by use of soft helmets, knee pads, softened environment
- Avoid contact sports, trampolines, three-wheelers
- Wear protective equipment appropriate to activity
- Regular visits to hemophilia treatment center for care
- Follow recommended immunization schedule
- Regular exercise to strengthen muscles and joints

Pharmacologic
- Intravenous plasma-free recombinant factor VIII for prophylaxis and treatment of bleeding episodes
- Intranasal desmopressin acetate (DDAVP) for minor bleeding with mild hemophilia
- Oral aminocaproic acid (Amicar) for clot stabilization before dental procedures
- Acetaminophen (Tylenol) for pain

Patient/Family Education
- Disease process
- Genetic implications
- Home factor administration
- Medication administration
- Strategies to prevent bleeding
- Exercise and activity plan

Outcomes and Follow-Up
- The child will experience minimal bleeding episodes.
- The child will receive recommended immunizations.
- The child will receive care at a hemophilia center.
- The child will engage in appropriate exercise and physical activity.

- The child will not develop inhibitor antibodies.
- The family will verbalize understanding of the disease process and genetic implications.
- The family will demonstrate intravenous factor administration.
- The family will demonstrate medication administration.
- The family will identify strategies to prevent bleeding.
- The family will recognize signs of bleeding episode.
- The family will demonstrate nonpharmacologic management of bleeding episodes.

LEUKEMIA

Description
Leukemia is cancer of the blood-forming tissues. The main types of leukemia seen in children are acute lymphoblastic leukemia (ALL) and acute myeloid leukemia (AML).

Etiology
In leukemia, the blood-forming tissues produce large numbers of immature white blood cells called blasts. These blast cells infiltrate body tissues, especially highly vascular areas, and crowd out normal cells by competing for nutrients. Infiltration of the bone marrow causes decreased numbers of red blood cells, white blood cells, and platelets. The accompanying increased pressure within the marrow produces bone pain and bone weakening. Infiltration of the lymph glands, spleen, and liver leads to enlargement and fibrosis. With central nervous system infiltration there is increased intracranial pressure and possibly cranial nerve involvement. Additional sites of infiltration are the kidneys, testes, prostate, ovaries, gastrointestinal tract, and lungs.

Incidence and Demographics
- Incidence can be found in Table 14–2.
- Leukemia is the most common childhood cancer, and 25.5% of childhood cancer deaths are due to leukemia. The cure rate for ALL is about 90%; for AML, 40%–45%. The incidence of ALL is higher in White children than in Black children, but after the age of 3 years, the incidence of AML is higher in Black children.

Risk Factors
- Ionizing radiation
- Benzene
- Down syndrome
- Fanconi anemia
- Diamond-Blackfan syndrome
- Li-Fraumeni syndrome

Table 14-2. Incidence of Childhood Leukemia per 100,000

	<1 year	1–4 years	5–9 years	10–14 years	15–19 years
Leukemia	4.2	8.7	3.8	2.8	2.8
ALL	1.9	7.4	3.1	1.8	1.6
AML	1.3	0.9	0.4	0.6	0.8

Prevention and Screening
- No prevention or screening indicated

Assessment

History
- Bone pain
- Bleeding gums
- Pallor
- Bruising and petechiae
- Fatigue and lethargy
- Fever
- Frequent infections

Physical Exam
- Swollen lymph glands
- Hepatosplenomegaly
- Chloromas
- Testicular enlargement
- Anterior mediastinal mass

Diagnostic Studies
- Complete blood count
- Variable white blood cell count: an initial count >50,000/mm3 places child in a less-favorable prognostic category (high risk)
- Bone marrow aspiration for definitive diagnosis

Management

Invasive
- Bone marrow transplant
  - ALL during second remission
  - AML during first remission

Nonpharmacologic
- Strategies to deal with side effects of chemotherapy
- Infection prevention
- Balance of rest and activity

Pharmacologic
- Pharmacologic treatment can be found in Table 14–3
- Patient/family education
  - Disease process and treatment plan
  - Strategies to deal with side effects of chemotherapy
  - Infection prevention
  - Rest and activity

Table 14-3. Pharmacologic Treatment for Leukemia, by Phase

Phase	ALL	AML
Induction of remission	4 wks chemotherapy • Prednisone or dexamethasone • Vincristine • L-asparaginase • Doxorubincin for high-risk only > 95% remission rate	2 courses (6–8 wks each) • Cytarabin • Doxorubicin • Etoposide or thioguanine About 75% remission rate
Central nervous system preventive therapy	Intrathecal methotrexate Cranial radiation for only high-risk	Intrathecal cytarabine No cranial radiation
Consolidation	Various combinations with intensity and duration based on risk	Stem cell transplant
Maintenance	Oral 6-mercaptopurine and methotrexate for 2.5–3 years	No maintenance therapy

Outcomes and Follow-Up
- The child will attain and maintain remission.
- The child will experience minimal side effects of chemotherapy.
- The child will maintain a balance of rest and activity.
- The family will integrate strategies to deal with side effects of chemotherapy.
- The family will practice infection prevention.
- The child will experience monitoring for potential long-term effects of treatment:
  - Testing for cognitive delay
  - Growth monitoring for pituitary dysfunction
  - Monitoring for reproductive dysfunction
  - Complete blood counts to identify secondary neoplasms
  - Electrocardiography or echocardiography to detect cardiomyopathy
  - Liver function studies
  - Dental exams

HODGKIN'S DISEASE

Description
Hodgkin's disease is a cancer that originates in the lymphoid system, involves primarily the lymph nodes, and spreads through the lymphatic system.

Etiology
The specific cause of Hodgkin's disease is unknown, but research suggests that an abnormal immune response to an infectious agent, possibly the Epstein-Barr virus, may have a role in the development of the disease. In most cases, the disease starts in the B lymphocytes. Staging is based on systemic symptoms, number of sites, location of involved lymph nodes above or below diaphragm, and presence of extranodal involvement.

Incidence and Demographics

Hodgkin's disease is responsible for only 1% of deaths due to childhood cancer. More than 80% of people with newly diagnosed disease will be long-term survivors.

The incidence of Hodgkin's disease in children can be found in Table 14–4.

Risk Factors

- Human immunodeficiency virus (HIV) infection
- Family history
- Epstein-Barr viral infection
- Compromised immune system

Prevention and Screening

- No prevention or screening indicated

Assessment

History

- Fever
- Night sweats
- Weight loss
- Pruritus
- Anorexia
- Nausea

Physical Exam

- Swollen lymph nodes above the diaphragm, commonly the cervical, supraclavicular, and axillary areas
- Nodes are firm, nontender, and movable

Diagnostic Studies Also Used for Staging

- Biopsy of lymph nodes shows Reed-Sternberg cells, an abnormal type of B lymphocytes
- Chest radiography
- CT scan
- Positron emission tomography with contrast (FDG-PET)
- Complete blood count
- Erythrocyte sedimentation rate
- Serum electrolytes
- Renal and liver function tests
- Serum albumin and serum lactate dehydrogenase
- Bone marrow aspiration

Table 14-4. Incidence of Hodgkin's Disease in Children

5–9 year olds	10–14 year olds	15–19 year olds
0.4 per 100,000	1.1 per 100,000	3.1 per 100,000

Management

Invasive

- Autologous stem cell transplantation (ASCT)

Nonpharmacologic

- Radiation therapy

Pharmacologic

CHEMOTHERAPY: COMBINATION ABVD
- Doxorubicin (Adriamycin)
- Bleomycin (Blenoxane)
- Vinblastine (Velban)
- Dacarbazine (DTIC-Dome)

Patient/Family Education

- Disease process and treatment plan
- Common side effects of treatment

Outcomes and Follow-Up

- The child will experience full remission.
- The child will show evidence of adequate rest during treatment.
- The child will attend school as much as possible.
- The child and family will verbalize understanding of diseases process and treatment plan.
- The child and family will demonstrate strategies to cope with side effects of treatment.

REFERENCES

Anderson, N. (2006). Hydroxyurea therapy: Improving the lives of patients with sickle cell disease. *Pediatric Nursing, 32,* 541–543.

Ansell, S. M., & Armitage, J. O. (2006). Management of Hodgkin lymphoma. *Mayo Clinic Proceedings, 81,* 419–426.

Belson, M., Kingsley, B., & Holmes, A. (2007). Risk factors for acute leukemia in children: A review. *Environmental Health Perspectives, 115,* 138–145.

Brown, P. (2006). Answers to key questions about childhood leukemia—for the generalist. *Contemporary Pediatrics, 23,* 81–98.

Centers for Disease Control and Prevention. (2004). *United States cancer statistics.* Retrieved from http://apps.nccd.cdc.gov/uscs/Table.aspx?Group=TableChild&Year=2004&Display=n

Cheng, J., & Sakamoto, K. M. (2005). *Topics in pediatric leukemia—acute myeloid leukemia.* Retrieved from http://www.medscape.com/viewarticle/498646

Curry, H. (2004). Bleeding disorder basics. *Pediatric Nursing, 30,* 402–405, 428–429.

Fosdal, M. B., & Wojner-Alexandrov, A. W. (2007). Events of hospitalization among children with sickle cell disease. *Journal of Pediatric Nursing, 22,* 342–346.

Hockenberry, M. J., & Wilson, D. (2007). *Wong's nursing care of infants and children.* St. Louis, MO: Mosby Elsevier.

Killip, S., Bennett, J. M., & Chambers, M. D. (2007). Iron deficiency anemia. *American Family Physician, 75,* 671–678.

Lindsey, T., Watts-Tate, N., Southwood, E., Routhieaux, J., Beatty, J., Calamaras, D., et al. (2005). Chronic blood transfusion therapy practices to treat strokes in children with sickle cell disease. *Journal of the American Academy of Nurse Practitioners, 17,* 277–282.

Mehta, S. R., Afenyi-Annan, A., Byrns, P. J., & Lottenberg, R. (2006). Opportunities to improve outcomes in sickle cell disease. *American Family Physician, 74,* 303–310.

National Institutes of Health. (2002). *The management of sickle cell disease.* Retrieved from http://www.nhlbi.nih.gov/health/prof/blood/sickle/sc_mngt.pdf

Panepinto, J. A., & Brousseau, D. C. (2005). Acute idiopathic thrombocytopenic purpura of childhood—diagnosis and therapy. *Pediatric Emergency Care, 21,* 691–695.

Pruthi, R. K. (2005). Hemophilia: A practical approach to genetic testing. *Mayo Clinic Proceedings, 80,* 1485–1499.

Robertson, J., & Shilkofski, N. (Eds.). (2005). *The Harriet Lane handbook.* Philadelphia: Mosby.

Sherry, D. D. (2008). Avoiding the impact of musculoskeletal pain on quality of life in children with hemophilia. *Orthopaedic Nursing, 27,* 103–108.

Sur, D. K., & Bukont, E. L. (2007). Evaluating fever of unidentifiable source in young children. *American Family Physician, 75,* 1805–1811.

U. S. Preventive Services Task Force. (2006). *Screening and supplementation for iron deficiency anemia.* Retrieved from http://www.ahrq.gov/clinic/uspstf/uspsiron.htm

U. S. Preventive Services Task Force. (2007). *Screening for sickle cell disease in newborns.* Retrieved from http://www.ahrq.gov/clinic/uspstf/usphemo.htm

15

Immunologic Disorders

Clara J. Richardson, MSN, RN-BC

HUMAN IMMUNODEFICIENCY VIRUS (HIV)/
ACQUIRED IMMUNODEFICIENCY SYNDROME (AIDS)

Description

Human immunodeficiency virus (HIV) is the organism that causes acquired immunodeficiency syndrome (AIDS), a chronic disease of the immune system.

Etiology

HIV is transmitted by contact with another person's infected blood, body fluids, or secretions. The virus then binds to the CD4 receptor on the cell membrane of the T-lymphocytes. The DNA of the virus joins the T-cell DNA and is reproduced as the T-cell replicates, a process called reverse transcription. The result is suppression of cell-mediated immunity. Immediately after infection, the virus is disseminated throughout the lymphoid organs. The speed of progression from HIV infection to AIDS is variable. The diagnosis of AIDS is based on an extremely low CD4 cell count and development of AIDS-defining illnesses.

Incidence and Demographics

The incidence of HIV/AIDS in children under the age of 13 years is 0.1 per 100,000 in the United States. Of these children, approximately 79% are Black, 10% are White, 8% are Hispanic, and 3% are Asian. Perinatal transmission is the major route of transmission for this age group.

The time from HIV diagnosis to development of AIDS can be found in Table 15–1.

Risk Factors

- Maternal HIV infection, injection drug use, sexual partner with injection drug user
- Human blood product recipient in areas without adequate product screening
- Maternal HIV infection
- Injection drug use
- Sexual partner with HIV infection
- Sexual partner with injection drug use
- Human blood product recipient in areas without adequate product screening

Prevention and Screening

- Prevention by decreasing risk of maternal transmission
  - Antiretroviral therapy for pregnant women with HIV
  - Cesarean section delivery
  - Limit time between rupture of fetal membranes and delivery to under 4 hours
  - Avoid breastfeeding
- Screening of pregnant women for HIV allows prevention and early treatment for infected infants
- Screening of newborns at risk for maternal transmission

Assessment

History

- Chronic or recurrent diarrhea
- Growth failure
- Frequent infections
- Developmental delay

Physical Exam

- Swollen lymph glands
- Hepatosplenomegaly
- Oral candidiasis
- Inflammation of the parotid gland

Table 15–1. Time to Development of AIDS From HIV Diagnosis

Age (years)	≥12 months	<12 months
<13	88%	12%
13–14	54%	46%
15–19	81%	19%

- AIDS-defining conditions:
  - *Pneumocystis carinii* pneumonia: Life-threatening fungal lung infection
  - Lymphoid interstitial pneumonitis: Infiltration of alveoli and interstitial spaces with mature lymphocytes
  - Recurrent bacterial infections
  - HIV encephalopathy: Impaired brain growth, cognitive impairment, loss of developmental milestones
  - Cytomegalovirus disease: Viral infection causing retinitis, death of retinal cells
  - *Mycobacterium avium-intracellulare complex* infection
  - Pulmonary or esophageal candidiasis: Yeast infection
  - Herpes simplex disease: Viral infection with painful skin eruptions
  - Cryptosporidiosis: Parasitic infection causing diarrhea

Diagnostic Studies
- CD4+ (helper T-cell) counts and percentages
  - <200 or 14% of lymphocytes indicative of AIDS
  - Monitored every 3–4 months
- Positive HIV antibody test (ELISA) for children 18 months of age or older
- Repeat positive HIV DNA polymerase chain reaction (PCR) survey
- Positive HIV RNA assay: Monitored every 3–4 months
- Positive viral load test

Management
Invasive
- No invasive management indicated

Nonpharmacologic
- Healthy diet
- Balance of rest and activity

Pharmacologic
- Age for initiation of treatment depends on CD4, HIV RNA, and symptoms for children 1 year of age and older
- All HIV-positive infants (less than 12 months old) should be treated
- Highly active antiretroviral therapy (HAART) for children should include at least three drugs in at least two classes
  NUCLEOSIDE REVERSE TRANSCRIPTASE INHIBITORS (NRTIS) PREMATURELY END DNA REPLICATION
  - Abacavir
  - Lamivudine
  - Emtricitabine
  - Didanosine
  - Zidovudine
  - Stavudine

NONNUCLEOSIDE REVERSE TRANSCRIPTASE INHIBITORS (NNRTIS) INHIBIT REVERSE TRANSCRIPTASE
- Efavirenz
- Nevirapine

PROTEASE INHIBITORS (PIS) INHIBIT VIRAL REPLICATION LATER IN PROCESS
- Lopinavir/ritonavir
- Fosamprenavir

- Trimethoprim/sulfamethoxazole (TMP/SMX): Bactrim, Septra prophylaxis for *Pneumocystis carinii*
- Isoniazid or rifampin prophylaxis for *Mycobacterium tuberculosis* with positive skin test or TB contact
- Clarithromycin or azithromycin prophylaxis for *Mycobacterium avium-cellulare complex*
- VZIG prophylaxis for varicella-zoster virus with exposure
- Recommended immunization schedule:
  - Measles-mumps-rubella (MMR) depending on symptoms and CD4 cell count
  - Varicella vaccine: Same considerations
  - 23-valent pneumococcal polysaccharide vaccine (PPS23) at ages 2 and 5 years
  - Annual influenza virus vaccine

Patient/Family Education
- Disease process and treatment plan
- Transmission and prevention
- Implications of lab results
- Medication regimen and implications of noncompliance
- Nutrition
- Balance of rest and activity
- Prevention and signs of opportunistic infections
- Community resources
- Advocacy: social stigma, rights

Outcomes and Follow-Up
- The child will experience balance of rest and activity.
- The child will maintain healthy diet as evidenced by adequate growth.
- The child will attain age-appropriate developmental milestones.
- The child will receive recommended well-child care.
- The child will not experience social stigma related to HIV status.
- The family will verbalize understanding of disease process and treatment plan.
- The family will demonstrate strategies to prevent transmission of HIV.
- The family will verbalize understanding of lab results.
- The family will maintain strict adherence to medication regimen.
- The family will demonstrate strategies to prevent opportunistic infections.
- The family will recognize signs and seek prompt treatment of opportunistic infections.
- The family will actively advocate within healthcare system, childcare setting, school system, and community to ensure child's rights.

SYSTEMIC ALLERGIC REACTIONS

Description
Systemic allergic reaction, anaphylaxis, is the body's acute-onset, potentially fatal response to an allergen.

Etiology
IgE is synthesized upon exposure to an allergen and becomes fixed on mast cells and basophils. Mast cells and basophils release histamine and other mediators of inflammation, causing vasodilation, bronchoconstriction, and increased capillary permeability. Fluid leaks into the interstitial spaces with reduced arterial pressure and rapid onset of symptoms.

Common allergens in children include:

Foods
- Cow's milk
- Eggs
- Peanuts and tree nuts
- Fish and shellfish
- Wheat, soy, or sesame
- Citrus fruits, strawberries
- Chocolate

Drugs and Medical Products
- Drugs
- Contrast media
- Latex
- Blood products

Venom
- Hymenoptera (bees, wasps)
- Snakes
- Jellyfish
- Spiders

Incidence and Demographics
The incidence of anaphylaxis is not known, but several trends have been identified. The incidence seems to be increasing based on emergency room statistics. Anaphylaxis occurs more commonly in community settings than in healthcare settings, and the largest number of occurrences is in children and adolescents.

Risk Factors
- Positive allergen skin test
- Elevated quantitative allergen-specific IgE level
- Recent insect stings
- Concurrent asthma

Prevention and Screening
- Prevention consists of avoiding allergen exposure
- Screening to identify allergen may be done with allergen skin testing and quantitative allergen-specific IgE levels

Assessment
History
- Exposure to allergen

Physical Exam
- Skin
  - Itching
  - Flushing
  - Hives
  - Angioedema
- Respiratory
  - Cough
  - Dyspnea
  - Hoarseness
  - Stridor
  - Wheezing
- Gastrointestinal
  - Nausea
  - Vomiting
  - Diarrhea
  - Abdominal pain
- Cardiovascular
  - Dizziness
  - Hypotension
  - Shock
  - Incontinence
- Headache

Diagnostic Studies
- Plasma histamine within 15–60 minutes of onset
- Serum or plasma tryptase within 15–180 minutes of onset

Management
Invasive
- No invasive management indicated

Nonpharmacologic
- Establish airway
- Oxygen
- Trendelenburg position with hypotension

Pharmacologic
- Epinephrine
- Albuterol
- Diphenhydramine (Benadryl)
- Methylprednisolone (Solu-Medrol)
- Intravenous normal saline

Patient/Family Education
- Description and treatment of anaphylaxis
- Avoidance strategies
- Use of Epi-Pen
- Emergency action plan

Outcomes and Follow-Up
- The child will receive prompt treatment of anaphylaxis.
- The child will maintain open airway and adequate circulation.
- The child will experience relief of symptoms.
- The child will wear medical alert jewelry.
- The child will have an Epi-Pen available at all times.
- The child and family will identify allergens.
- The child and family will practice avoidance strategies.
- The family will verbalize understanding of anaphylaxis.
- The family will demonstrate use of Epi-Pen.
- The family will develop emergency action plan for childcare, school, extracurricular activities.

SYSTEMIC LUPUS ERYTHEMATOSUS

Description
Systemic lupus erythematosus (SLE) is a chronic, autoimmune, inflammatory disease affecting multiple body systems and is characterized by exacerbations and remissions.

Etiology
The exact mechanism of SLE initial onset is not completely known. It is thought that predisposing factors such as genetic factors, sex hormones, and environmental triggers interact to initiate a disordered immune response. Environmental triggers that are being investigated include sun exposure, infection, and drugs. The immune response is characterized by activated helper T-cells that stimulate B-cells to cause secretion of auto-antibodies and immune complex. The immune complexes are deposited in kidney, brain, heart, spleen, lung, gastrointestinal, skin, and peritoneum tissues. The final result is organ disease and death.

Incidence and Demographics
Approximately 1.5 million people in the United States have SLE, with only 15%–20% diagnosed during childhood. The peak incidence in children is between 11 and 15 years of age. Asian-American, Black, Native American, and Hispanic children have a higher incidence. When compared with adults with SLE, children have more severe disease at onset, more organ involvement, and a more aggressive clinical course.

Risk Factors
• Family history of autoimmune diseases

Drugs That May Cause SLE That Resolves When the Drug Is Discontinued
• Hydralazine (Apresoline)
• Procainamide (Procanbid)
• Isoniazid (INH)
• Chlorpromazine (Thorazine)
• Phenytoin (Dilantin)
• Carbamazepine (Tegretol)

Prevention and Screening
• There is no known prevention and no screening is indicated

Assessment
History
• Recurrent fevers
• Fatigue
• Weight loss

Physical Exam (Must Have at Least Four of the Eleven American College of Rheumatology Classification Criteria for Diagnosis)
• Arthritis with pain and swelling of two or more peripheral joints
• Malar (cheek) rash
• Renal disorder with proteinuria or cellular casts
• Neurologic disorder with seizures or psychosis
• Hematologic disorder with hemolytic anemia, leukopenia, lymphopenia, or thrombocytopenia
• Immunologic disorder with positive LE cell preparation, anti-DNA antibodies, anti-Sm antibodies, or false-positive serologic test for syphilis
• Disc-shaped rash: Red, scaling patches
• Positive antinuclear antibody (ANA)
• Photosensitivity
• Mouth or nose ulcers
• Serositis: Pleuritis or pericarditis

Diagnostic Studies
• Complete blood count
• Urinalysis
• Antinuclear antibody
• Autoantibodies

Management
Invasive
- No invasive management indicated

Nonpharmacologic
- Strategies to prevent coronary artery disease
  - Avoid smoking
  - Maintain healthy weight
  - Healthy diet
  - Monitor blood pressure, cholesterol, lipids
- Strategies to prevent infection
- Strategies to prevent osteoporosis
  - Exercise and physical activity
  - Diet fortified with calcium and vitamin D
- Strategies to limit sun exposure to minimize photosensitive rash

Pharmacologic
- Corticosteroids: Prednisone for anti-inflammatory and immunosuppressive properties
- Antimalarial drugs: Hydroxychloroquine (Plaquenil) for rash and musculoskeletal symptoms
- Immunosuppressive drugs:
  - Azathioprine (Imuran) for nephritis
  - Cyclophosphamide (Cytoxan) for renal and central nervous system involvement
- Calcium and vitamin D supplements to prevent osteoporosis with corticosteroids
- Nonsteroidal anti-inflammatory drugs (NSAIDs) for arthritis:
  - Naproxen
  - Ibuprofen
- Antihypertensive agents:
  - Diuretics (Lasix)
  - Angiotensin-converting enzyme inhibitors (Captopril, Enalapril, Lisinopril)
  - Calcium channel blockers (CCBs): Procardia

Patient/Family Education
- Disease process and treatment plan
- Medication administration
- Strategies to prevent coronary artery disease, infection, osteoporosis, sun exposure

Outcomes and Follow-Up
- The child will experience minimal exacerbations of the disease.
- The child will experience minimal side effects of drug therapy.
- The child will experience balanced activity and rest.
- The child and family will verbalize understanding of disease process and treatment plan.
- The child and family will integrate strategies to prevent coronary artery disease, infection, osteoporosis, and sun exposure.
- The family will demonstrate effective medication administration.

REFERENCES

Centers for Disease Control and Prevention. (2007). *HIV/AIDS surveillance report.* Retrieved from
http://www.cdc.gov/hiv/topics/surveillance/resources/reports/#surveillance

Hiraki, L. T., Benseler, S. M., Tyrrell, P. N., Hebert, D., Harvery, E., & Silverman, E. D. (2008). Clinical
and laboratory characteristics and long-term outcome of pediatric systemic lupus erythematosus.
The Journal of Pediatrics, 152, 550–556.

Hockenberry, M. J., & Wilson, D. (2007). *Wong's nursing care of infants and children.* St. Louis, MO:
Mosby Elsevier.

Plowfield, L. A. (2007). HIV disease in children 25 years later. *Pediatric Nursing, 33,* 274–278.

Pongmarutani, T., Alpert, P. T., & Miller, S. K. (2006). Pediatric systemic lupus erythematosus:
Management issues in primary practice. *Journal of the American Academy of Nurse Practitioners,
18,* 258–267.

Robertson, J., & Shilkofski, N. (Eds.). (2005). *The Harriet Lane handbook.* Philadelphia: Mosby.

Simons, F. E. R. (2008). Anaphylaxis. *Journal of Allergy and Clinical Immunology, 121,* S402–S407.

Working Group on Antiretroviral Therapy. (2008). *Guidelines for the use of antiretroviral agents in
pediatric HIV infection.* Retrieved from http://AIDSinfo.nih.gov/contentfiles/PediatricGuidelines/pdf

16

Neuromuscular Disorders

Clara J. Richardson, MSN, RN-BC

NEURAL TUBE DEFECTS

Description

Neural tube defects (NTD) are malformations of the spinal cord, brain, and vertebrae. The main NTDs are encephalocele, anencephaly, and spina bifida. Encephalocele is an opening in the skull that allows a portion of the brain to protrude. In anencephaly, there is no brain development above the brainstem. The most common NTD is spina bifida, which takes three forms. Spina bifida occulta is nonvisible separation in the vertebrae. Meningocele is a vertebral defect with a visible protruding sac filled with spinal fluid. The third, more serious form is myelomeningocele, in which the protruding sac contains portions of spinal cord.

Etiology

The neural groove of the fetus folds to become the neural tube, which develops into the spinal cord and vertebral arches by 26 days. A neural tube defects develops if the groove does not close completely. Although the cause remains uncertain, genetic and environmental factors have been identified.

Incidence and Demographics

In the United States, the incidence of encephalocele is 10 in 100,000 births, of anencephaly 20 in 100,000, and of myelomeningocele 60 in 100,000. The prevalence is much higher in Ireland and Wales, and much lower in Africa. Females are affected more often except in sacral NTDs, which have an equal occurrence. A higher incidence has also been noted with increased maternal age and with lower socioeconomic level.

Risk Factors

- Folic acid deficiency
- Some chromosomal disorders
- Maternal use of certain medications
    - Valproic acid (Depakene, Depakote)
    - Carbamazepine (Tegretol)
    - Isotretinoin (Accutane)
- Maternal exposure to toxic solvents
    - Benzene
    - Carbon tetrachloride
    - Trichloroethylene
- Maternal excessive alcohol use
- Maternal exposure to hyperthermia (sauna, high fever)
- Maternal prepregnancy obesity
- Past history of child with NTD multiplies recurrence risk by 30

Prevention and Screening

- Enrichment of grain products with folic acid
- Use of multivitamin containing folic acid for all women of childbearing age
- Screening by measurement of alpha-fetoprotein (AFP) in maternal blood
    - At 16–18 weeks gestation
    - If elevated, further diagnostic testing is indicated

Assessment of a Child With Myelomeningocele

History

- History of a sibling with NTD

Physical Exam: Variable Depending on Location and Severity of Defect

- Neurological:
    - Motor paralysis and sensory loss below the level of the defect
    - Chiari malformation with defect above sacral area
        · Brainstem and part of cerebellum displaced downward toward neck
        · Spinal cord compression causes difficulty swallowing, choking, apnea, stiff arms, opisthotonos position, sleep disorders
    - Hydrocephalus
    - Seizure disorder
    - Strabismus

- Cognitive:
  - Mild cognitive disability in 25% of children
  - Learning disability
  - Impaired organizational ability
  - Impaired motor response, memory, hand function
  - Attention-deficit hyperactivity disorder
- Musculoskeletal:
  - Delayed rolling over, sitting, walking
  - Joint deformities
  - Pathological fractures
  - Spinal curvatures
- Bowel and bladder:
  - Incomplete bladder emptying
  - Urine incontinence
  - Constipation or diarrhea
  - Fecal incontinence
- Skin irritation or decubitus ulcers on weight-bearing body surfaces
- Latex allergy
- Obesity
- Sexual issues
  - Uncontrolled erections and retrograde ejaculations in males
  - Decreased genital sensation and lubrication in females
  - Precocious puberty in females

Diagnostic Studies
- High resolution ultrasound to detect specific anomaly
- Amniocentesis to measure AFP and acetylcholinesterase (ACH), substances found in fetal cerebrospinal fluid, for definitive diagnosis
- CT scan, MRI, ultrasound at birth to detect sac contents

Management
Invasive
- The benefits of prenatal surgical repair have not been proven to outweigh the risks of the procedure at this time
- Delivery by cesarean section to prevent damage of the sac
- Surgical closure of the defect within the first few days of life
- Surgical placement of ventricular shunt to treat hydrocephalus
- Spinal surgery to allow more brainstem room with Chiari malformation
- Vesicostomy to form opening through abdominal wall and into bladder
- Creation of an artificial urinary sphincter to drain urine from bladder
- Bladder augmentation to increase bladder capacity
- Appendicovesicostomy in which the appendix is used to connect bladder to abdominal wall
- Adenoidectomy for child with sleep apnea

Nonpharmacologic

PREOPERATIVE
- Prone position with hips and legs slightly flexed
- Cover sac with sterile, saline-moistened dressing
- Infant warmer

POSTOPERATIVE
- Prone or side position
- Daily head circumference to detect hydrocephalus

ONGOING
- Early intervention program beginning in infancy
- Braces, splints, walker, wheelchair for mobility
- Daily intermittent urinary clean catheterization
- Bowel training program
- Padding to prevent skin irritation
- Continuous positive airway pressure (CPAP) or bilevel positive airway pressure (BiPAP) for sleep disorder
- Weight control with diet and exercise
- Latex precautions
- Penile implant, injection, or prostaglandin prior to sexual intercourse
- Vaginal lubrication prior to intercourse

Pharmacologic
- Antibiotics to treat or prevent central nervous system infection
- Pain management during postoperative period
- Long-term prophylactic oral antibiotics to prevent urinary tract infections
  - Cephalexin (Keflex)
  - Trimethoprim/sulfamethoxazole (Bactrim, Septra)
- Medications to enhance bladder function
  - Oxybutynin chloride (Ditropan)
  - Pseudoephedrine (Sudafed)
  - Imipramine (Tofranil)
- Medications to enhance bowel function
  - Laxatives such as lactulose, MiraLax, senna, bisacodyl
  - Fiber supplement such as psyllium (Metamucil)
  - Saline enemas
- Leuprolide (Lupron) for precocious puberty

Patient/Family Education
- Treatment plan
- Surgical procedures
- Complications
- Importance of early intervention
- Strategies to promote attainment of developmental skills

- Skin care
- Bowel and bladder training
- Items containing latex
- Nutrition and weight control
- Medication administration

Outcomes and Follow-Up
Preoperative
- The child will not experience spinal cord infection.
- The child's exposed spinal cord and nerves will not be physically injured.
- The child will maintain adequate body temperature.
- The family will verbalize understanding of surgical procedures and treatment plan.

Postoperative
- The child will experience healing of incision.
- The child will experience effective pain management.

Ongoing
- The child will participate in an early intervention program beginning in infancy.
- The child will maintain intact skin integrity.
- The child will exhibit adequate growth.
- The child will attain normal developmental milestones.
- The child will not develop a latex allergy.
- The child will experience prompt treatment of complications.
- The child and family will manage adaptive equipment to promote mobility.
- The child and family will manage equipment for bladder and bowel function.
- The family will identify signs of complications.
- The family will demonstrate safe, effective medication administration.

HYDROCEPHALUS

Description
Hydrocephalus is an accumulation of excess cerebrospinal fluid (CSF) in the ventricles of the brain. The disorder is classified as congenital when it is the result of neural tube defects or developmental malformation of the brain. It is classified as acquired when the cause is infection, hemorrhage, or tumor.

Etiology
Excess accumulation of CSF occurs when there is a flow obstruction, noncommunicating hydrocephalus, or impaired absorption in communicating hydrocephalus. The ventricles enlarge, the skull expands, and the brain thins and atrophies.

Incidence and Demographics
The incidence of congenital hydrocephalus is 4 in every 1,000 live births.

Risk Factors
- Neural tube defects
- Meningitis
- Traumatic head injury
- Brain tumor
- Prematurity with intraventricular or subarachnoid hemorrhage
- Prenatal infections such as toxoplasmosis, cytomegalovirus, rubella

Prevention and Screening
- Folic acid supplements for all women of childbearing age
- Prompt treatment of meningitis, head injury, brain tumor, complications of prematurity, prenatal infections
- Screening by evaluation of physical signs

Assessment
History
- Preterm birth
- Neural tube defect
- Brain malformation
- Brain tumor
- Head injury
- Physical signs

Physical Exam
INFANTS
- Irritability
- Poor feeding
- Tense, bulging fontanel
- Increased head circumference
- Decreased level of consciousness
- Slow papillary reaction
- Sunset eyes with sclera visible above iris
- Seizures
- Preterm infants with hydrocephalus due to hemorrhage may show only a gradual increase in head circumference without other manifestations

OLDER CHILDREN
- Morning headache
- Nausea and vomiting
- Decreased level of consciousness
- Urinary incontinence
- Seizures
- Visual disturbances

Diagnostic Studies
- Ultrasound in prenatal period or infancy
- CT scan
- MRI

Management
Invasive
- Surgical placement of ventriculoperitoneal shunt to drain excess CSF
- Shunt revisions due to child's growth, or shunt infection or malfunction
- Endoscopic third ventriculostomy
  - Small opening made in floor of third ventricle
  - For noncommunicating hydrocephalus
- Surgical removal of causes of obstruction

Nonpharmacologic
PREOPERATIVE
- Elevate head of bed for untreated hydrocephalus
- Daily head circumference

POSTOPERATIVE
- Flat position on nonoperative side
- Raise head of bed gradually
- Support head and neck
- Incision care

Pharmacologic
- Acetazolamide (Diamox) for slowly progressing communicating hydrocephalus
- Pain management after surgical procedures

Patient/Family Education
- Treatment plan
- Care of incision after surgical procedure
- Signs of shunt infection
- Signs of shunt malfunction
- Shunt exposure to MRI may alter programmed settings and should be avoided if possible; the neurosurgeon may need to reprogram after unavoidable exposure

Outcomes and Follow-Up
- The child will experience effective pain management.
- The family will verbalize understanding of treatment plan.
- The family will demonstrate incision care after surgical procedure.
- The family will identify signs of shunt infection or malfunction:
  - Drainage, odor, tenderness, swelling at incision site
  - Fever
  - Headache with progressive worsening
  - Nausea or vomiting
  - Abdominal pain
  - Behavioral change such as irritability, drowsiness, change in school performance, change in level of consciousness
  - Sunset eyes or visual disturbance
  - Tense, bulging fontanel in infants
  - Loss of developmental milestones

SEIZURES

Description
A seizure is an excessive, synchronized discharge of cortical neurons causing a change in motor, sensory, or cognitive function. Seizure disorder, or epilepsy, is defined as multiple seizures not precipitated by a known cause. The term status epilepticus refers to a prolonged seizure lasting at least 30 minutes. Seizures are classified by focus and physical signs.

Etiology
Seizures may be caused by acute illness, toxin ingestion, central nervous system infection, or traumatic brain injury.

Incidence and Demographics
As many as 1 in 10 children will experience at least one seizure. Children with seizure disorders have a higher incidence of attention deficit/hyperactivity disorder, learning disability, anxiety disorder, and depression than children with other chronic diseases.

Risk Factors
- Cerebral palsy
- Autistic spectrum disorder
- Inborn error of metabolism
- Progressive neurologic disorder

Prevention and Screening
Prevention strategies include prompt treatment for infections, prevention of head injury, fever care. Screening involves evaluation of physical signs.

Assessment
History
- Changes in behavior on the previous day
- Unusual sleep pattern on the prior evening or morning
- Exposure to possible precipitating factors such as infection, trauma, drugs, ingested substances

Physical Exam
- See classification section below

Diagnostic Studies
- Complete blood count and lumbar puncture to rule out infection
- Serum toxin screens for suspected ingestions
- Electroencephalogram (EEG) to classify seizure type
- CT scan or MRI to rule out physical causes
- PET scan to show brain metabolic activity and SPECT scan to map brain blood flow before surgery
- Newer tests include magnetoencephalography (MEG) and functional MRI (fMRI) to show seizure focus and metabolic changes in the brain
- Routine blood studies such as drug levels, complete blood counts, and liver function tests to monitor effectiveness of antiepileptic drugs

Classification of Seizures

- Partial seizures account for 60% of seizure disorders in children. They have one focal area and often start with an aura and/or an abrupt change in behavior.
  - Simple partial seizures may have sensory sensations or local motor symptoms, but no loss of consciousness
  - Complex partial seizures (previously called psychomotor) have impaired consciousness, sensory sensations, purposeless movements, amnesia for event, sleepiness after event
  - Partial seizures evolving into secondary generalized seizures

Generalized Seizures

- Absence seizures (petit mal) are characterized by a brief loss of consciousness with minimal alteration in muscle tone
- Myoclonic seizures involve brief contraction of muscles with or without loss of consciousness
- Clonic seizures consist of violent jerking movements, excess salivation, incontinence of urine and stool
- Tonic seizures involve eye rolling, loss of consciousness, stiffening, apnea, shrill cry
- Tonic-clonic seizures (grand mal) consist of both tonic and clonic phases; the seizure is followed by semiconsciousness, visual and speech difficulty, impaired fine motor movement, confusion, vomiting, headache, amnesia for event
- Atonic seizures (akinetic or drop attacks) have momentary loss of muscle tone and consciousness causing child to fall

Special Seizure Syndromes

- Febrile seizures occur in about 5% of children between 6 months and 5 years, are provoked by fever, consist of tonic or clonic movement, and are not considered a seizure disorder
- Neonatal seizures are symptomatic of acute brain disorder and may have tonic, clonic, myoclonic, or subtle movements
- Infantile spasms occur during the first 4 to 8 months of life with brief muscle contraction, eye rolling, preceded by vocalization, possibly loss of consciousness

Management

Invasive

- Surgical removal of the seizure focus to cure seizure disorder
- Hemispherectomy, removal of one side of the brain, is a more drastic cure
- Corpus callosotomy, cutting the area that connects the two sides of the brain, is a palliative procedure
- Electrical stimulation of the vagus nerve with a subcutaneous devise is also palliative

Nonpharmacologic

- During seizure, position child safely on side, loosen clothing around neck, avoid restraint or inserting anything in mouth
- Ketogenic diet, high in fat and low in carbohydrates, has been shown to be effective in treating intractable seizures without medication
- Regular sleep appropriate for age
- Infection prevention and fever control
- Multivitamin supplement

Pharmacologic
- Phenytoin (Dilantin) for tonic-clonic or partial seizures, or status epilepticus
- Fosphenytoin (Cerebyx) for same indications as phenytoin
- Phenobarbital (Luminal) for neonatal, tonic-clonic, prolonged febrile seizures
- Carbamazepine (Tegretol, Carbatrol) for partial motor, partial complex, tonic-clonic seizures
- Oxcarbazepine (Trileptal) for partial seizures
- Valproic acid (Depakote, Depakene) for myoclonic, tonic, atonic, absence, tonic-clonic, and partial-onset seizures
- Ethosuximide (Zarontin) for absence, partial, and tonic-clonic seizures
- Lamotrigine (Lamictal) for absence, atonic, myoclonic, and tonic seizures and infantile spasms
- Felbamate (Felbatol) for partial seizures and infantile spasms
- Topiramate (Topamax) for partial-onset and tonic-clonic seizures and infantile spasms
- Gabapentin (Neurontin) for partial, myoclonic, and absence seizures
- Levetiracetam (Keppra) for partial seizures in adolescents
- Tiagabine (Gabitril) for partial seizures in adolescents
- Zonisamide (Zonegran) for partial and generalized seizures

Patient/Family Education
- Care during seizure
- Medication administration
- Common side effects of antiepileptic drugs such as sleepiness, decreased attention and memory, dysphasia, ataxia, visual disturbance, cognitive impairment
- Nonpharmacologic management strategies

Outcomes and Follow-Up
- The child will experience reduction in seizures or freedom from seizures.
- The child will experience prompt attention for signs of infection or fever.
- The child will establish regular sleep pattern and healthy diet.
- The child will experience minimal antiepileptic drug side effects.
- The child will not experience progressive cognitive and behavioral impairments due to seizure activity.
- The child will participate in activities appropriate for developmental level, avoiding heavy contact sports or unusually risky activities such as rock climbing.
- The family will demonstrate care during seizure.
- The family will demonstrate safe medication administration.
- The family will identify side effects of antiepileptic drugs.
- The family will provide supervision for bathing or swimming.
- The family will develop individualized plan of care with school nurse.
- The family will investigate state driving restrictions for adolescents with seizures.

CEREBRAL PALSY

Description
Cerebral palsy is a nonprogressive central nervous system disorder of movement and posture.

Etiology
This disorder is due to a brain injury or a genetically based problem with brain development.

Incidence and Demographics
The prevalence of cerebral palsy is about 2.0–2.5 per 1,000 children. Premature infants account for 40%–50% of cases. Associated problems include cognitive disability, visual impairment, hearing impairment, speech disorders, seizures, feeding and growth abnormalities, and behavioral/emotional disorders.

Risk Factors
- Premature birth
- Birth asphyxia
- Congenital brain malformation
- Coagulation abnormalities
- Complications of multiple gestation and intrauterine infection
- Small for gestational age
- Kernicterus as a result of hyperbilirubinemia

Prevention and Screening
Prevention strategy includes effective obstetrical care. Ultrasound is useful screening for brain malformations.

Assessment
History
- Delayed motor development
- Easily fatigued
- Frequent respiratory infections
- Constipation

Physical Exam
- Poor muscle control
- Poor balance
- Weakness
- Spastic, hypertonicity
- Hypotonicity during first few months of life
- Exaggerated reflexes
- Persistent primitive reflexes
- Asymmetrical reflex response
- Drooling

- Dental caries
- Atypical, involuntary movements (dyskinesias)
- Slow, writhing movements (chorea)
- Rigid posturing of head and neck (dystonia)
- Wide-based, unsteady gait
- Scissoring of legs or toe-walking position of feet
- Difficulty controlling hand and arm muscles during reaching

Diagnostic Studies
- CT scans and MRI
- Positron emission tomography (PET)
- Single photon emission computed tomography (SPECT)
- Diffusion tensor imaging (DTI)
- Swallowing studies for feeding difficulty

Management

INVASIVE
- Selective dorsal rhizotomy to permanently reduce leg spasticity
- Tendon lengthening to release contractures
- Tendon transfer to correct asymmetrical muscle tone

NONPHARMACOLOGIC
- Speech, occupational (OT), and physical therapy (PT)
- Neurodevelopmental therapy focusing on motor function
- Bracing, splinting, standing tables, positioning devices to maintain range of motion, prevent contractures, provide stability, control involuntary movements, and prevent osteoporosis
- Adaptive equipment such as crutches, walkers, canes, wheelchairs to maximize mobility
- Assistive technology such as self-care devices, computers to promote independence

PHARMACOLOGIC
- Nerve blocks, motor point blocks, and botulinum toxin (Botox) to decrease spasticity
- Oral medications to control movement:
  - Carbidopa-levodopa (Sinemet)
  - Trihexyphenidyl (Artane)
  - Diazepam (Valium)
  - Baclofen
  - Dantrolene (Dantrium)
  - Lorazepam (Ativan)
  - Clonazepam (Klonopin)
- Intrathecal baclofen therapy delivered into the spinal fluid with an implanted pump

PATIENT/FAMILY EDUCATION
- Explanation of disorder and treatment plan
- Therapeutic strategies (PT, OT, speech, etc.)
- Strategies to promote effective eating and swallowing
- Skin care with adaptive equipment, splints, braces, positioning devices
- Assistive technology
- Communication strategies
- Medication administration

Outcomes and Follow-Up
- The child will participate in an early intervention program.
- The child will receive prompt intervention for associated problems (hearing, vision, etc.).
- The child will utilize adaptive equipment effectively.
- The child will utilize assistive technology.
- The child will develop effective communication.
- The child will maintain intact skin.
- The child will demonstrate adequate growth.
- The child will participate in a variety of environments, including home, school, child care, and neighborhood settings.
- The family will verbalize understanding of the disorder and treatment plan.
- The family will utilize variety of professional disciplines to determine therapy plan.
- The family will demonstrate medication administration.

MUSCULAR DYSTROPHY

Description
Duchenne muscular dystrophy is an X-linked recessive, progressive skeletal muscle disorder and the most common form of muscular dystrophy in children.

Etiology
The disorder is caused by a genetic mutation in the dystrophin gene which causes an absence of dystrophin, a protein necessary for skeletal and cardiac muscle stability. Without dystrophin, there is an inflammatory process in the muscles that causes progressive necrosis of muscle fibers.

Incidence and Demographics
The incidence is 1 in 3,000 male births. Muscle weakness is usually noticed by age 3–4 years. Affected boys are usually unable to walk by early adolescence. Respiratory failure or cardiomyopathy often causes death in the early to mid-20s. With long-term ventilation, some young men are living into their 30s and 40s.

Risk Factors
Family history in about two-thirds of cases.

Prevention and Screening
No prevention or screening indicated.

Assessment

History of Progressive Deterioration
- Delayed walking
- Frequent tripping, falls

Physical Exam
- Muscle weakness starting with hip girdle muscles
- Walking on tiptoes or waddling gait
- Difficulty getting up from supine position on floor
- Hypertrophy of calf muscles
- Contractures
- Spinal curvatures
- Mild cognitive impairment
- Respiratory failure
- Cardiomyopathy

Diagnostic Studies
- Elevated serum creatinine phosphokinase (CPK)
- Muscle biopsy shows decreased dystrophin levels and fatty infiltration
- Electromyography (EMG) shows decreased muscle potential
- Radiography to monitor spinal changes

Management

Invasive
- Possible tendon lengthening to release contractures

Nonpharmacologic
- Physical and occupational therapy
- Range of motion
- Adaptive equipment such as braces, walkers, wheelchairs
- Noninvasive ventilation (NIV) for sleep-related upper airway obstruction and chronic respiratory insufficiency
- Intermittent positive pressure breathing (IPPB), CPAP, mechanical in-exsufflator to mimic cough
- Psychologist or psychiatrist as needed

Pharmacologic
- Corticosteroid therapy to slow progression of muscle weakness
- Antibiotics to treat infection

Patient/Family Education
- Disease progression and treatment plan
- Medication administration
- Adaptive equipment
- Use of respiratory devices
- Nutritional modifications
- Exercise program
- Care options such as home care, respite care, nursing facility care

Outcomes and Follow-Up
- The child will demonstrate use of adaptive equipment.
- The child will maintain intact skin.
- The child will receive adequate nutrition.
- The child will participate in activity and exercise as tolerated.
- The child will participate in self-care as able.
- The child and family will verbalize understanding of disease progression and treatment plan.
- The child and family will choose care setting.
- The child and family will discuss quality of life concerns and end-of-life care.
- The child and family will not experience social isolation.
- The child and family will utilize a variety of professional disciplines to cope with physical and emotional needs.
- The family will demonstrate use of respiratory devices and medication administration.

MENINGITIS

Description
Meningitis is inflammation of the meninges that cover the brain and spinal cord.

Etiology
Meningitis may be caused by bacteria or viruses. The most common causes of bacterial meningitis in neonates are group B streptococci, *Listeria monocytogenes*, and *Escherichia coli*. In older children, *Streptococcus pneumoniae* and *Neisseria meningitides* are the common causes. Meningitis usually follows invasion of the bloodstream by the causative organism. The organism then penetrates the blood–brain barrier and reaches the subarachnoid space.

Incidence and Demographics
The incidence of neonatal meningitis is about 2–10 cases per 10,000 live births. Meningitis is more common in Native Americans, Inuits, and Blacks. Since the introduction of the *Haemophilus influenzae* type b vaccine in 1987, the incidence of bacterial meningitis has declined by more than 99%. The pneumococcal vaccine was introduced in 2000 and the incidence of meningitis caused by *Streptococcus pneumonia* has declined to 1.1 cases per 100,000. The incidence of *Neisseria meningitides* is 4 per 100,000 and should be decreasing as the use of meningococcal vaccine increases. Possible complications of meningitis include cerebral palsy, attention deficit/hyperactivity disorder, learning disorders, seizure disorders, deafness, blindness, and paralysis of facial or neck muscles. Meningococcemia may lead to septic shock, disseminated intravascular coagulation, and has a 90% mortality rate.

Risk Factors
- Crowded living conditions
- Poor living conditions

Prevention and Screening
Prevention involves immunizations against causative organisms and effective treatment of bacterial infections. Pregnant women should be treated with ampicillin or penicillin for group B streptococcal infection. No widespread screening is indicated.

Assessment
History
- Maternal infection during pregnancy
- Infection of the nasopharynx, sinuses, middle ear
- Severe head trauma with a skull fracture
- Penetrating wound

Physical Exam
- Fever, chills
- Vomiting
- Severe headache
- Photophobia
- Nuchal rigidity
- Irritability, confusion, lethargy
- Positive Kernig sign: Pain when knee flexed then extended in supine position
- Positive Brudzinski sign: Involuntary hip or knee flexion when head flexed while lying in supine position
- Petechial or purpuric rash and joint pain with *Neisseria meningitides*
- Infants have more general signs
  - Change in feeding habits
  - Vomiting
  - Seizure
  - Irritability, altered level of consciousness, high-pitched cry

Diagnostic Studies
- Lumbar puncture (see Table 16–1)
- A new test (Xpert EV) on cerebrospinal fluid can help distinguish viral from bacterial meningitis in about $2^1/_2$ hours
- Causative organism may be identified with culture of cerebrospinal fluid (CSF), blood, or throat

Management
Invasive
- No invasive management indicated

Table 16–1. Lumbar Puncture Diagnostic Test

	Normal CSF	Bacterial	Viral
Color	Clear	Cloudy	Slightly cloudy or clear
WBC lymphs	0–5	High with increased polys	Slightly high with increased
Protein	10–30	Elevated	Normal or slightly elevated
Glucose	40–80	Decreased	Normal

Nonpharmacologic
- Respiratory isolation until completion of 24 hours of antimicrobial therapy
- Decrease environmental stimuli, specifically noise and lighting
- Position for comfort with head of bed slightly raised
- Support of ventilation as needed
- Restriction of fluid intake as needed

Pharmacologic
- Neonates:
  - Ampicillin and cefotaxime (Claforan)
  - Flucloxacillin (Nafcillin)
  - Vancomycin (Vancocin) and ceftazidime (Fortaz)
- 1–3-months:
  - Ampicillin and cefotaxime
  - Ceftriaxone (Rocephin)
- 3 months–5 years:
  - Cefotaxime
  - Ceftriaxone
- Older than 5 years:
  - Cefotaxime or ceftriaxone and
  - Vancomycin
- Pain management
- Antipyretics and anticonvulsants as needed
- Intravenous therapy to maintain fluid and electrolyte balance

Patient/Family Education
- Disease process and treatment plan
- Prevention by immunization

Outcomes and Follow-Up
- The child will verbalize comfort of position and environment.
- The child will experience effective pain management.
- The child will receive prompt treatment for fever and seizures.
- The child will show signs of adequate hydration without fluid overload.
- The child will recover without long-term complications.
- The family will verbalize understanding of disease and treatment plan.
- The family will provide immunizations to all family members.

ENCEPHALITIS

Description
Encephalitis is an inflammatory process of the central nervous system caused by a variety of viruses, bacteria, fungus, and parasites.

Etiology
Viruses are the main causative agent of encephalitis in children. The virus may directly invade the central nervous system, cross the blood-brain barrier from another site of infection, or be transmitted from mosquito vectors. The result is inflammation, edema, and neuronal cell death. The prevalent cause in children is herpes simplex.

Incidence and Demographics
Herpes simplex encephalitis is uncommon, but children account for 30% of the cases.

Risk Factors
- Maternal infection during pregnancy
- Living in mosquito-infested areas

Prevention and Screening
- Effective treatment for maternal infection during pregnancy

Assessment
History
- Nausea and vomiting
- Headache
- Dizziness

Physical Exam
- Altered level of consciousness
- Focal seizures
- Fever
- Lethargy
- Neck stiffness
- Ataxia or tremors

Diagnostic Studies
- CT scan
- MRI
- Culture from CSF, blood, nose, throat, urine

Management
Invasive
- Possibly intracranial pressure monitoring

Nonpharmacologic
- Decrease environmental stimuli, specifically noise and lighting
- Position for comfort with head of bed slightly raised

Pharmacologic
- Acyclovir for herpes simplex
- Antiepileptics for seizures
- Antipyretics for fever
- Pain management

Patient/Family Education
- Disease process and treatment plan
- Potential long-term complications

Outcomes and Follow-Up
- The child will experience effective pain management.
- The child will receive prompt treatment for fever and seizures.
- The child will show signs of adequate hydration without fluid overload.
- The child will recover without neurologic, functional, or cognitive impairment.
- The family will verbalize understanding of disease and treatment plan.

BRAIN TUMORS

Description
Brain tumors are solid tumors originating from glial cells, nerve cells, epithelial cells, blood vessels, pineal gland, or hypophysis. Major childhood brain tumors, in order of prevalence, include astrocytoma, medulloblastoma, cerebellar astrocytoma, brainstem glioma, and ependymoma.

Etiology
The cause of brain tumors is unknown.

Incidence and Demographics
In 2004, the incidence of brain and other nervous system cancer was 4 per 100,000 in children younger than 1 year old; 4.1 between ages 1 and 4 years; 3.3 between 5 and 9 years; 2.5 between 10 and 14 years; and 2.2 between 15 and 19 years. These cancers accounted for 25% of total deaths due to childhood cancer.

Risk Factors
- Exposure to vinyl chloride has been associated with increased incidence of gliomas
- Ionizing radiation is a rare cause of primary brain tumors
- Genetic disorders such as Li-Fraumeni syndrome, retinoblastoma

Prevention and Screening
- No prevention or screening indicated

Assessment
History
- Headache that is worse in the morning
- Vomiting that is worse in the morning and not related to eating
- Irritability, fatigue

Physical Exam

NEUROMUSCULAR CHANGES
- Clumsiness, loss of balance
- Weakness, poor fine motor control
- Hypo- or hyperactive reflexes
- Spasticity or paralysis
- Positive Babinski sign

VITAL SIGNS
- Decreased pulse and respiratory rates
- Increased blood pressure
- Decreased pulse pressure
- Hypo- or hyperthermia

CRANIAL NERVE NEUROPATHY
- Head tilt
- Visual disturbances

OTHER SIGNS
- Seizures
- Tense, bulging fontanel
- Nuchal rigidity
- Papilledema

Diagnostic Studies
- CT scan
- MRI

Management
Invasive
- Surgical resection of as much of tumor as possible
- Lasers to destroy tumor tissue
- Possible shunt placement for hydrocephalus

Nonpharmacologic
- Radiation therapy to shrink tumor
- Cooling blanket for hyperthermia after brain surgery
- Postoperative position determined by surgery
  - Nonoperative side
  - Infratentorial procedure: Flat and side-lying
  - Supratentorial procedure: Head elevated above heart level
- Postoperative saline eye drops if swelling prevents eye closure

Pharmacologic
- Chemotherapy
  - Carmustine
  - Lomustine
  - Vincristine
  - Cisplatin
  - Carboplatin
  - Etoposide
  - Thiotepa
  - Cyclophosphamide
- Corticosteroids or diuretics for brain edema
- Antiepileptics for seizures
- Pain management

Patient/Family Education
- Disease process and treatment plan
- Postoperative care
- Side effects of radiation and chemotherapy
- Care of residual problems
- Medication administration

Outcomes and Follow-Up
- The child will return to usual activities and school as soon as possible.
- The child will wear a helmet for active play or sports until skull is healed.
- The child will adhere to activity restrictions.
- The child will experience minimal residual problems such as growth retardation; cranial nerve palsies; and cognitive, sensory, or motor impairment.
- The child and family will verbalize understanding of disease process and treatment plan.

HEAD INJURIES

Description
Head injury is trauma from impact and inertia forces that cause a broad spectrum of injury; the results range from full recovery to severe functional disability.

Etiology
The causes of head injury in children are numerable and include motor vehicle, pedestrian, and bicycle accidents; falls; near-drowning; sports injuries; attempted suicide; and physical abuse. Head injury is the result of two forces, impact and inertia. Impact is when the head hits a surface or is struck by a moving object. Impact forces can cause scalp injury, skull fracture, contusion, or epidural hematoma. Inertia forces occur when the brain moves within the skull, tearing nerves and blood vessels. Concussion, diffuse injury, and subdural hematomas are the result of inertia forces.

Incidence and Demographics

About 1 in 25 children receive medical attention for head injury. Approximately 1 in 500 experiences a change in their level of consciousness, which is considered traumatic brain injury, the most common cause of acquired disability in children. Head injuries occur more often in the spring and summer, on weekends, and in the afternoon.

Risk Factors

- Children from birth to age 5 years
- Adolescents
- Conduct disorder
- Attention-deficit hyperactivity disorder
- Prematurity
- Young parents
- Unstable family dynamics

Prevention and Screening

- Many head injuries are preventable and screening involves evaluation after an injury
    - Effective restraint of children in motor vehicles with car seats, booster seats, air bags, and position in the rear seat
    - Driver education, night curfews, graduated licensing for adolescents
    - Reduced speed limits and physical separation of pedestrians and traffic in areas frequented by children
    - Bicycle and motorcycle helmets
    - Protective equipment for sports and recreation activities
    - Playground and water safety

Assessment

History

- Very specific description of injury

Physical Exam

- Lethargy, confusion, irritability
- Loss of consciousness
- Severe headache
- Speech, vision, movement impairment
- Repeated vomiting
- Pupillary changes
- Bulging fontanel
- Retinal hemorrhage
- Respiratory difficulty
- Seizures
- Laceration or large bump on head
- CSF or blood in nasal or ear drainage

Diagnostic Studies
- CT scan
- MRI
- Radiographs

Management
Invasive
- Suture of lacerations or torn dura
- Surgical reduction of depressed skull fracture
- Orthopedic surgery for contractures

Nonpharmacologic
- Airway and oxygenation maintenance
- Spine stabilization
- Decreased environmental stimuli initially
- Play and activity therapy
- Physical, occupational, and speech therapy
- Adaptive equipment such as crutches, walkers, wheelchairs
- Enteral feeding if unable to eat
- Treatment of vision or hearing impairment
- Special education for cognitive impairment

Pharmacologic
- Intravenous therapy to maintain fluid and electrolyte balance
- Total parenteral nutrition with coma state
- Medication as needed for cerebral edema, pain, or seizures
- Antibiotics with lacerations or penetrating injury
- Medications to treat spasticity and rigidity:
  - Baclofen
  - Dantrolene (Dantrium)
  - Diazepam (Valium)
  - Botulinum toxin A (Botox)

Patient/Family Education
- Injury and treatment plan
- Strategies to regain impaired function and promote normal development
- Strategies to prevent future injury
- Medication administration
- Skin care with mobility impairment
- Use of adaptive equipment
- Alternative feeding techniques
- Utilization of various professional disciplines

Outcomes and Follow-Up
- The child will maintain open airway and adequate oxygenation.
- The child will not experience increased intracranial pressure.
- The child will maintain intact skin and full range of motion.
- The child will receive adequate nutrition.
- The child will recover without long-term complications.
- The child will utilize adaptive equipment for impaired function.
- The family will verbalize understanding of injury, treatment plan, and residual disability.
- The family will demonstrate strategies to regain function and promote normal development.
- The family will demonstrate use of adaptive equipment, skin care, alternative feeding techniques, and medication administration.
- The family will utilize a variety of professional disciplines.

SPINAL CORD INJURIES

Description
Spinal cord injuries are compression, contusion, laceration, and transection of the spinal cord. Long-term function depends on the level of the injury.

Etiology
Causes of spinal cord injury in children include motor vehicle crashes, birth injuries, lap belt injuries, sports injuries, and child abuse. Damage to the cord comes from cellular tissue damage, hemorrhage, inflammation, and edema.

Incidence and Demographics
Approximately 10,000 individuals sustain spinal cord injuries each year in the United States. Of these, 3%–5% occur in children under 15 years of age and 20% in individuals under age 20. In those over 5 years of age, spinal cord injuries are more prevalent in males. Complications of spinal cord injury in children are neurogenic bladder and bowel, pressure ulcers, autonomic dysreflexia, scoliosis, hip dysplasia, spasticity, hypercalcemia, latex allergy, pulmonary complications, and deep vein thrombosis (DVT).

Risk Factors
- Improper restraint in motor vehicles
- Skeletal dysplasias, juvenile rheumatoid arthritis, Down syndrome

Prevention and Screening
No screening indicated, but prevention involves:
- Safe restraint in motor vehicles with car seats and booster seats

Assessment

History
- Specific description of injury

Physical Exam
- Flaccid extremities
- Numbness, tingling, burning sensation
- Weakness or paralysis
- Priapism
- Incontinence of bladder or bowel
- Loss of rectal tone

Diagnostic Studies
- MRI

Management

Invasive
- Surgical decompression of cord with clot, herniated disc, or lesion
- Surgical intervention for scoliosis
- Tendon transfers to increase hand function
- Urinary diversion or bladder augmentation

Nonpharmacologic
- Cervical collar initially and spinal immobilization with brace for 1–2 months
- Bowel and bladder management
- Skin care and pressure ulcer prevention
- Prevention and management of autonomic dysreflexia
- Elevate head
- Loosen clothing
- Empty bladder
- Consistent bowel and bladder program
- Promotion of normal development
- Clean, intermittent catheterization for neurogenic bladder
- Bowel training program
- Physical and occupational therapy
- Possible lifelong ventilator support and/or phrenic nerve pacing for high cervical injury
- Patient-triggered synchronous intermittent mandatory ventilation (SIMV-assist/control mode) for midlevel injury
- Chest physical therapy to mobilize secretions
- DVT prophylaxis during first 12 months after injury
- Functional electrical stimulation to increase mobility of extremities and bowel and bladder function

Pharmacologic
- Possibly methylprednisolone (Solu-Medrol) to decrease inflammation
- Stool softeners or laxatives to promote regular bowel elimination
- Dicyclomine (Bentyl) to promote increased bladder capacity
- Antihypertensive medication for autonomic dysreflexia
- Baclofen or botulinum toxin type A (Botox) for spasticity
- Pamidronate (Aredia) for hypercalcemia
- Medication for chronic neuropathic pain
- Clonidine hydrochloride to improve ambulation with partial spinal cord injuries

Patient/Family Education
- Injury and treatment plan
- Bowel and bladder management strategies
- Skin care and prevention of pressure ulcers
- Prevention of latex allergy
- Use of adaptive equipment
- Signs of hypercalcemia:
    - Behavior changes, malaise, lethargy
    - Nausea, vomiting, abdominal pain
    - Polyuria, polydipsia, dehydration
- Signs of autonomic dysreflexia:
    - Headache
    - Profuse sweating, flushed skin
    - Blurred vision
    - Decreased rate
    - Increased blood pressure
    - Anxiety
    - Nasal congestion
- Use of respiratory equipment, chest physiotherapy (CPT)
- DVT prevention
- Medication administration
- Implications for development of sexuality

Outcomes and Follow-Up
- The child will maintain open airway and effective respiration.
- The child will maintain intact skin.
- The child will demonstrate adequate growth.
- The child will not develop latex allergy.
- The child will demonstrate effective bowel and bladder elimination.
- The child and family will utilize adaptive devices.
- The child will participate in a variety of environments including home, school, child care, and neighborhood settings.
- The family will verbalize understanding of injury and treatment plan.
- The family will identify signs of autonomic dysreflexia and hypercalcemia.
- The family will demonstrate strategies to prevent autonomic dysreflexia and DVT.
- The family will utilize a variety of professional disciplines to determine therapy plan.
- The family will demonstrate medication administration.
- The family will discuss sexuality as the child matures.

LYME DISEASE

Description
Lyme disease is a tick-borne disorder caused by a spirochete, *Borrelia burgdorferi*.

Etiology
The spirochete enters the skin through the bite of an infected deer tick and is disseminated through the blood and lymphatic systems.

Incidence and Demographics
Lyme disease commonly occurs in the New England, Middle Atlantic, Upper Midwest, and Pacific Northwest states. The peak season is April through October.

Risk Factors
- Exposure to ticks
- Inadequate protection

Prevention and Screening
- Prevention:
  - Light-colored clothing
  - Long-sleeved shirt tucked into pants
  - Long pants tucked into socks
  - Avoid weedy, grassy areas
  - Cautious use of insect repellent
- Screening involves careful bare skin check for ticks after outside activity in suspect areas

Assessment
History
- History of tick bite or outside activity in suspect area

Physical Exam
EARLY LOCALIZED DISEASE
- Appears between 3 and 32 days after exposure
- Erythema migrans (small red papule enlarging to form a ring with a red, raised border with a clear center) in 70%–80% of cases
- Fever, headache, muscle aches, malaise

EARLY DISSEMINATED DISEASE
- Appears 3–10 weeks after exposure
- Multiple, smaller, secondary erythema migrans
- Systemic symptoms mentioned above
- Anorexia, stiff neck, lymphadenopathy, splenomegaly, conjunctivitis, sore throat, abdominal pain, cough
- 1% develop carditis

LATE DISEASE
- Intermittent, recurrent symptoms up to 12 months after exposure
- Arthritis of large joints
- Peripheral neuropathy
- Encephalopathy

Diagnostic Studies
- Immunoassay for B. *burgdorferi*-specific IgM at 3–4 weeks
- Immunoassay for B. *burgdorferi*-specific IgG after several weeks to months
- Lumbar puncture will show Lyme disease–specific antibodies with CNS involvement

Management
Invasive
- No invasive management indicated

Nonpharmacologic
- Comfort measures

Pharmacologic
- Doxycycline (Vibramycin) for children 8 years and older
- Amoxicillin (Amoxil) for younger children
- Ceftriaxone (Rocephin) or penicillin for arthritis, carditis, CNS involvement

Patient/Family Education
- Disease process and treatment plan
- Medication administration
- Prevention of exposure to ticks

Outcomes and Follow-Up
- The child will complete entire course of antibiotic therapy.
- The child will recover without arthritis, carditis, or CNS involvement.
- The child and family will identify strategies to prevent future exposure.
- The family will verbalize understanding of disease process and treatment plan.
- The family will demonstrate medication administration.

REFERENCES

Batshaw, M. L., Pellegrino, L., & Roizen, N. J. (2007). *Children with disabilities*. Baltimore: Paul H. Brookes.

Buckner, J. C., Brown, P. D., O'Neill, B. P., Meyer, F. B., Wetmore, C. J., & Uhm, J. H. (2007). Central nervous system tumors. *Mayo Clinic Proceedings, 82*, 1271–1286.

Centers for Disease Control and Prevention. (2004). *United States cancer statistics*. Retrieved from http://apps.nccd.cdc.gov/uscs/Table.aspx?Group=TableChild&Year=2004&Display=n

Centers for Disease Control and Prevention. (2009). *Learn about lyme disease*. Retrieved from http://www.cdc.gov/ncidod/dvbid/lyme/index.htm

Gaudreault, N. Gravel, D., Nadeau, S., & Houde, S. (2005). Motor function in Duchenne muscular dystrophy children: A review of the literature. *Critical Reviews in Physical and Rehabilitation Medicine, 17*, 231–248.

Hockenberry, M. J., & Wilson, D. (2007). *Wong's nursing care of infants and children*. St. Louis, MO: Mosby Elsevier.

Jones, M. W., Morgan, E., & Shelton, J. E. (2007). Primary care of the child with cerebral palsy: A review of systems. *Journal of Pediatric Health Care, 21*, 226–237.

Lomax-Bream, L. E. (2007). The impact of spina bifida on development across the first 3 years. *Developmental Neuropsychology, 31*, 1–20.

Lovering, R. M., Porter, N. C., & Block, R. J. (2005). The muscular dystrophies: From genes to therapies. *Physical Therapy, 85*, 1372–1388.

Partap, S., & Fisher, P. G. (2007). Update on new treatments and developments in childhood brain tumors. *Current Opinion in Pediatrics, 19*, 670–674.

Robertson, J., & Shilkofski, N. (Eds.). (2005). *The Harriet Lane handbook*. Philadelphia: Mosby.

Rudy, C. (2005). Questions and answers. *Journal of Pediatric Health Care, 19*, 127–128.

Saez-Llorens, X., & McCracken, G. H. (2003). Bacterial meningitis in children. *Lancet, 361*, 2139–2148.

Sejvar, J. J., Kohl, K. S., Bilynsky, R., Blumberg, D., Cvetkovich, T., Galama, J., et al. (2007). Encephalitis, myelitis, and acute disseminated encephalomyelitis (ADEM): Case definitions and guidelines for collection, analysis, and presentation of immunization safety data. *Vaccine, 25*, 5771–5792.

Simonds, A. K. (2006). Recent advances in respiratory care for neuromuscular disease. *Chest, 130*, 1879–1886.

Simpkins, C. J. (2005). Ventriculoperitoneal shunt infections in patients with hydrocephalus. *Pediatric Nursing, 31*, 457–462.

Stevens, P. M. (2006). Lower limb orthotic management of Duchenne muscular dystrophy: A literature review. *Journal of Prosthetics and Orthotics, 18*, 111–119.

Tobias, N., Mason, D., Lutkenhoff, M., Stoops, M., & Ferguson, D. (2008). Management principles of organic causes of childhood constipation. *Journal of Pediatric Health Care, 22*, 12–23.

Vogel, L. C., Hickey, K. J., Klass, S. J., & Anderson, C. J. (2004). Unique issues in pediatric spinal cord injury. *Orthopaedic Nursing, 23*, 300–308.

Yaffe, S. J., & Aranda, J. V. (2005). *Neonatal and pediatric pharmacology: Therapeutic principles in practice*. Philadelphia: Lippincott, Williams, & Wilkins.

17

Musculoskeletal Disorders

Clara J. Richardson, MSN, RN-BC

DEVELOPMENTAL DYSPLASIA OF THE HIP (DDH)/
CONGENITAL DISLOCATED HIP (CDH)

Description
Developmental dysplasia of the hip (DDH), previously referred to as congenital dislocated hip, is the abnormal anatomical relationship between the femoral head and the acetabulum. The degree of dysplasia may be described as preluxation, subluxation, or dislocation. In preluxation, also called acetabular dysplasia, the acetabulum is shallow and the head of the femur remains in place. In hip subluxation the femoral head still makes contact with a part of the acetabulum, but is not in its normal position. The head of the femur makes no contact with the acetabulum in the dislocated hip.

Etiology
- The hip joint structures are fully formed by 11–12 weeks gestation. Dislocations occurring at this time are often associated with other neuromuscular conditions.
- In most cases, the hip joint is initially normal and then becomes abnormal (see risk factors).

Incidence and Demographics

- Approximately 1 child in 1,000 births is born with a dislocated hip and 10 in 1,000 with hip subluxation
- Among children with DDH, up to 60% are female, up to 50% had breech presentations, and up to 33% have a positive family history
- The left hip alone is affected in about 60% of cases, the right hip in 20%, and both hips in 20%

Risk Factors

- Female gender
- First-born status
- Positive family history
- Breech position
- Oligohydramnios, a decrease in amount of amniotic fluid
- The majority of children with DDH have no identifiable risk factors

Prevention and Screening

- There is no identified prevention for DDH and screening has become controversial.
- Traditionally newborns and infants up to 3 months of age have been screened with the Ortolani and Barlow tests. With the child in supine position, the hips are flexed to 90° while the knees also are flexed. The examiner places middle fingers over the greater trochanters and thumbs on the inner thighs and tests each hip independently. To perform the Ortolani test, the examiner gently abducts the hip while applying forward pressure on the trochanter and then backward pressure from the thumbs. With a positive Ortolani a palpable "clunk" is noted as the femur head slips back into the acetabulum. This test is performed only by a trained nurse practitioner or physician.
- The Barlow test is done with the infant in the same position, but the hips are adducted and downward pressure is applied with a palpable "clunk" noted in a positive Barlow. This test is performed only by a trained nurse practitioner or physician.
- Infants with positive signs have then been further screened by ultrasound at 2 weeks of age.
- In 60%–80% of newborns with abnormal hips on screening, the condition resolves spontaneously by 2–8 weeks of age.
- 90% of newborns showing abnormal hips on ultrasound have spontaneous resolution between 6 weeks and 6 months.
- In 2006, the U.S. Preventative Task Force concluded that there is insufficient evidence for routine DDH screening.
- The American Academy of Pediatrics recommends serial clinical examination of hips, hip imaging for female infants born breech, and optional hip imaging for breech males or females with positive family histories.

Assessment

- History of risk factors
- Physical exam
  - Positive Galeazzi sign: unequal knee height when infant is in supine position with knees flexed and hips adducted
  - Asymmetry of gluteal thigh skin folds

- Limited hip abduction by 3 months of age
  - Delayed walking
  - Limping or walking on toes
  - Waddling gait
  - External rotation of leg
- Diagnostic studies
  - Ultrasound in infants between 6 weeks and 6 months to identify degree of dysplasia and document hip stability during treatment
  - Radiographs after 4 to 6 months of age to show relationship between the femoral head and the femur

Management
- Pavlik harness for infants up to 6 months with reducible dislocations
  - Harness has chest, shoulder, anterior and posterior stirrup straps to keep hips flexed and in abduction, but allow some movement
  - Usually worn continuously for 6 weeks, then part-time for 6 more weeks
  - If unable to maintain femoral head placement at 2 to 3 weeks, treatment discontinued
- Hip spica cast for failed Pavlik treatment or in children older than 6 months
  - Applied after closed or open reduction
  - Worn for about 12 weeks
- Patient/family education

Care of Infant in Pavlik Harness
- Importance of keeping harness on, but also instructions on reapplication in case harness is removed
- Undershirts under harness to protect skin and clothes over harness to keep it clean
- Check for skin irritation 2–3 times each day
- Avoid lotion, powder, and cream under harness
- Positioning for feeding and car travel
- Promoting normal development

Care of Infant in Hip Spica Cast
- Keep cast clean and dry with moisture barrier
- Frequent diaper changes
- Padding edges of cast to prevent skin irritation
- Positioning for feeding and car travel
- Promoting normal development

Outcomes and Follow-Up
- The child will not experience complications of treatment such as skin breakdown, femoral nerve palsy, femoral head damage, avascular necrosis, or early onset osteoarthritis of the hip.
- The child will comply with regular follow-up visits until the end of skeletal growth.
- The family will verbalize understanding of the care and maintenance of the Pavlik harness or hip spica cast.

CONGENITAL CLUBFOOT

Description
Clubfoot, talipes equinovarus, is a congenital deformity of the foot with four main features. The forefoot is inverted and adducted, the heel turns inward (varus), the ankle turns downward (equines), and the leg is rotated internally.

Etiology
The exact etiology of clubfoot is unknown, but is considered to be multifactorial.

Incidence and Demographics
- The incidence of clubfoot is 1–2 per 1,000 live births
- The incidence is higher in Hispanics and Pacific Islanders and lower in Asians
- It is bilateral in approximately 50% of cases.

Risk Factors
- Male gender
- Positive family history

Assessment
- History of risk factors

Physical Exam
- Smaller foot with soft heel pad
- Concave medial border
- Convex lateral border
- Deep transverse plantar crease
- Internally rotated heel
- Tight Achilles tendon with limited dorsiflexion

Diagnostic Studies
- Prenatal ultrasound
- Radiographs to identify severity
- Periodic radiographs or ultrasounds to monitor effectiveness of treatment

Management
Ponseti Method
- Weekly gentle manipulation and stretching of foot
- Weekly application of two-part cast with one section covering toes to below knee and another section covering knee and thigh, with knee held at 90° angle for 4–8 weeks
- Percutaneous tendoachilles lengthening with local anesthesia to allow dorsiflexion of foot
- Last cast hyperabducting foot to 70° external rotation and 15° dorsiflexion
- After cast removal, corrective brace consisting of shoes with connecting bar that holds affected foot in hyperabducted position (Denis Browne splint)
- Brace worn full-time for 2–3 months and then at naps and night for 3–4 years

French Physical Therapy Method

- Continuous passive motion machine for up to 10 hours per day for first 12 weeks
- Physical therapy to stretch and stimulate muscles for 5 days per week for first 2 months
- Parents taught to continue physical therapy at home
- Splinting and taping until 2–3 years of age

Invasive Management

- At 6–12 months of age, after failure of nonsurgical methods
- Release of tight tendons with pin fixation
- Followed by casting for 2–3 months and corrective bracing

Patient/Family Education

- Defect and treatment protocol
- Positioning, bathing, skin care, clothing
- Neurovascular, skin, pain assessment
- Care of cast, splint, or corrective brace

Outcomes and Follow-Up

- The child will have a foot that is functional, mobile, and pain-free.
- The child will walk on the whole sole of the foot with the heel touching the floor.
- The family will verbalize understanding of the defect and treatment plan.
- The family will demonstrate positioning, bathing, skin care, and clothing adaptations.
- The family will demonstrate care of appliance or cast.
- The family will identify and report neurovascular, skin, or comfort changes.

FRACTURES/DISLOCATIONS

Description

There are four common types of bone fractures in children. Children's bones may bend up to 45° without breaking, but the bone straightens slowly, has some degree of deformity, and is called a bend fracture. A buckle, or torus, fracture consists of a raised projection. A greenstick fracture is an incomplete fracture. Complete fractures divide the bone into segments. Children may have a fracture or injury of the growth plate, the physis. Growth plate injuries may result in shortened limb length or bone deformities. Fractures are accompanied by muscle contraction, soft tissue contusion, and bleeding.

A dislocation involves abnormal position of bone ends in joint sockets.

Etiology

A bone fractures when it is subjected to more force than it can absorb. Fractures in children may occur during play, competitive sports, motor vehicle accidents, or physical maltreatment.

Dislocations occur when direct or twisting trauma to ligaments forces bone ends and joint sockets into abnormal positions.

Incidence and Demographics

Approximately 27% of girls and 42% of boys will have a fracture during childhood. Children most commonly sustain fractures of the wrist, elbow, and clavicle. Fractures of the femur, pelvis, and tibia are the most common lower-extremity fractures in children. Growth plate injury accounts for about 25% of skeletal injuries in children.

The most common dislocations in children include phalanges, shoulders, elbows, hips, and knees.

Risk Factors

- Participation in high-risk activities such as contact sports, skateboarding
- Overweight and obesity
- Poor nutrition, particularly protein, vitamin D, and calcium deficiencies
- Excess intake of carbonated soft drinks
- Tobacco and alcohol use
- First fracture at young age
- Chronic conditions such as Duchenne muscular dystrophy, cystic fibrosis, cerebral palsy, sickle cell disease
- Disorders involving impaired motor skills, poor balance, postural instability
- Medical treatment such as immunosuppressive therapy, chemotherapy, corticosteroids, radiotherapy
- Family history
- Prenatal history of maternal smoking, poor nutrition, prematurity, very low birth weight

Prevention and Screening

- Protective gear for sports
- Safe, supervised playgrounds
- Motor vehicle safety measures
- Regular weight-bearing exercise
- Accident prevention education
- Balanced diet, healthy body weight

Assessment

History

- Circumstances of injury: mechanism of injury, severity of trauma, description appropriate to injury, previous fractures or dislocations
- Possible physical abuse should be suspected in children with multiple fractures in various stages of healing, femur fractures in nonwalking children, midshaft ulna fractures, skull fractures, rib fractures, and scapula fractures
- Family history of fractures, birth history, associated medical conditions and medications
- Growth measurements
- Physical activity, safety measures
- Nutritional history
- Tobacco or alcohol use

Physical Exam
- Observable deformity such as breaks in skin, swelling, bruising
- Pain, specifically point of maximum tenderness
- Active and passive range of motion
- Neurovascular status including warmth, color, capillary refill, sensation
- Dislocations are characterized by pain, swelling, and joint immobility

Diagnostic Studies
- Radiographs, ultrasounds, CT scans
- Full radiographic skeletal survey or bone scan if physical maltreatment is suspected
- Growth plate injuries are graded I–V using the Salter-Harris system
- Dislocations

Management
Invasive
- Open reduction
- Internal or external fixation

Nonpharmacologic
- Traction
- Procedural sedation, closed reduction, and casting
- Splints, slings
- Elevation of extremities
- Dislocations are treated with mild sedation or local anesthesia, manual reduction, possibly immobilization followed by active range of motion

Pharmacologic
- Pain management
- Antispasmodics for muscle spasms

Patient/Family Education
- Cast care
- Pain management
- Signs of neurovascular compromise
- Safe ambulation with crutches, walkers, wheelchair
- Motor vehicle safely, specifically use of restraints
- Modifications of activities of daily living such as using toilet or bathing
- Injury-prevention strategies for play, sports, and motor vehicles
- Strategies to promote balanced nutrition, weight control, and exercise

Outcomes and Follow-Up
- The child's bone will heal without complications such as circulatory impairment, nerve injury, compartment syndrome, bone deformity, growth abnormalities, osteomyelitis, kidney stones, or pulmonary embolism.
- The child and family will verbalize understanding of cast care, pain management, signs of complications, safe ambulation, and activities of daily living.
- The child and family will verbalize understanding of injury prevention strategies.
- The child and family will verbalize understanding of healthy nutrition, weight management, and exercise.

LEGG-CALVÉ-PERTHES DISEASE (LCPD)

Description
Legg-Calvé-Perthes Disease (LCPD) is a hip disorder involving avascular necrosis of the femoral head.

Etiology
- The course of the disease process follows four stages.
- The initial cause is unknown, but leads to a temporary decrease in blood supply to the proximal femoral epiphysis, resulting in necrosis and flattening of the femoral head.
- The second stage is the fragmentation stage, with revascularization of the proximal femoral epiphysis and new bone formation.
- In the reossification, or healing stage, new bone is formed over an average of 4 years' time.
- The final stage involves either gradual remodeling of the femoral head or residual deformity.

Incidence and Demographics
- The incidence of LCPD is about 1 in 1,200 children.
- The incidence is higher in males by 5:1.
- Higher incidence is reported among Asians, Native Alaskans, and central Europeans; lower among Blacks.
- The peak onset is between the ages of 4 and 8 years.

Risk Factors
- These factors are considered contributing factors more than risk factors:
- Transient synovitis, inflammation of the synovial membrane
  - Trauma
  - Venous congestion
  - Hyperviscosity of the blood
  - Thrombophilia, increased risk of blood clots

Prevention and Screening
- No identified prevention
- Prompt evaluation of hip pain or limp in children

Assessment
History
- Vague history of mild trauma causing hip pain that resolved
- Pain of groin, thigh, or knee worsened by activity and relieved by rest
- Slow onset of a painful limp

Physical Exam
- Limited abduction of the hip
- Pain with motion
- Limp with walking
- Muscle atrophy as disease progresses
- Uneven limb lengths

Diagnostic Studies
- Radiographs to establish diagnosis and follow disease progression
- Bone scintigraphy and MRI
- Arthrography, invasive imaging done under general anesthesia, to determine the best position of femoral head for healing

Management
Invasive Management Consists of Three Surgical Options
- Femoral osteotomy with pinning to hold femoral head in place
- Pelvic osteotomy with pinning to provide better coverage of the femoral head
- A combination of these is indicated in severe cases
- Surgical reconstruction and containment allows return to usual activities in 3–4 months

Nonpharmacologic Management
- Initial rest and no weight-bearing
- Abduction traction to stretch surrounding muscles
- Progressively restoring mobility through physical therapy and aqua therapy
- Abduction bracing to maintain containment while allowing ambulation and motion of knee and ankle, but preventing weight-bearing on affected hip
- Abduction casting for the same purpose as bracin
- Conservative treatment may last for 2–4 years, but bracing allows near normal activity

Pharmacologic Management
- Anti-inflammatory medications
- Pain management

Patient/Family Education
- Stages of the disease process
- Treatment protocol
- Medication schedule
- Pain management
- Physical therapy plan
- Application and care of containment appliance
- Activity restrictions

Outcomes and Follow-Up
- The child will be comfortable with adequate pain management.
- The child's femoral head will be securely contained in the acetabulum until healing is complete.
- The child will have a pain-free hip with full mobility.
- The child will not experience complications such as collapse of femoral head, subluxation of capital epiphysis, or degenerative arthritis.
- The child and family will verbalize understanding of disease process and treatment protocol.
- The child and family will demonstrate application and care of containment device.
- The child and family will follow medication schedule, physical therapy, activity restrictions.

OSTEOMYELITIS

Description
Osteomyelitis is an inflammation of the bone caused by blood-borne bacteria.

Etiology
- Initial bacteremia may be caused by infection in another part of the body, puncture wound, open trauma, surgical contamination.
- Inflammatory process begins in the metaphyseal venous sinus with exudates that can exit the bone and move into adjacent soft tissue.
- In children, the infection is usually contained in the growth plate, but may move into the joint space in infants where blood vessels cross from growth plate to epiphysis.
- Osteomyelitis in neonates is most often due to Group B streptococcus, *Staphylococcus aureus*, or gram-negative rods.
- *Staphylococcus aureus* is the most frequent causative organism in infants and children.
- Infection may result in bone destruction, abscess formation, and accumulation of dead bone (sequestra).

Incidence and Demographics
- The incidence of osteomyelitis in children is less than 1 in 10,000 preteen children.
- The long bones, such as the tibia or femur, are the most common sites.

Risk Factors
- Organism that is virulent and/or present in large numbers
- Foreign body
- Bone injury
- Immunosuppression
- Malnutrition

Prevention and Screening
- Prompt effective treatment of bacterial infections
- Evaluation of unexplained bone pain accompanied by fever

Assessment
History
- Bacterial infection
- Puncture wound or open trauma
- Surgery

Physical Exam
- Bone pain with fever
- Soft tissue redness, warmth, swelling, tenderness
- Limited joint range of motion
- Pathological fracture due to presence of infection

Diagnostic Studies
- Elevated white blood cell count, platelet count, erythrocyte sedimentation rate (ESR), and C-reactive protein
- Positive bacterial cultures of blood, joint fluid, aspirated subperiosteal pus
- MRI to identify extent of infection
- CT to show bone changes, soft tissue swelling, or abscess
- Bone scan to locate multiple lesions or lesions in difficult to assess areas
- Ultrasound to detect bone changes, abscess, or joint effusion
- Radiographs show bone changes in 7–10 days

Management

Pharmacologic Management
- IV antibiotics until C-reactive protein returns to normal value, then oral antibiotics
- Nafcillin (Unipen), clindamycin (Cleocin), or oxacillin for *Staph. aureus*
- Vancomycin (Vancocin) for methicillin-resistant *Staph. aureus*
- Cefotaxime (Claforan), oxacillin, or gentamicin (Garamycin) for neonates
- Pain and fever management

Nonpharmacologic Management
- Position for comfort with support of affected extremity
- Avoid weight-bearing until healing well underway
- Physical therapy to restore function
- Increased calorie diet to compensate for decreased appetite
- Assess extremity for circulation, sensation, pain

Invasive Management
- Surgical debridement if infection does not respond to treatment within 36 hours or to manage bone damage
- Evacuate purulent material before the periosteum is destroyed
- Remove sequestra with chronic infection
- May be followed by irrigation with antibiotic solution for up to 48 hours

Patient/Family Education
- Treatment protocol
- Mobility restrictions
- Medication administration

Outcomes and Follow-Up
- The child will be comfortable with adequate pain management.
- The child will have fully functional extremity with minimal bone damage.
- The child and family will verbalize understanding of, and adhere to, treatment protocol.
- The child and family will demonstrate correct use of mobility devises such as crutches or wheelchair.

JUVENILE IDIOPATHIC ARTHRITIS (JIA)

Description
Juvenile idiopathic arthritis (JIA) is a chronic inflammatory disease of the joints with onset before 16 years of age. This disorder was previously called juvenile rheumatoid arthritis (JRA).

Etiology
- Idiopathic
- Inflammation of the synovium, the lining of the joints, causes the synovium to produce excess fluid
- Effusion and joint erosion develop
- The inflammation spreads and can damage cartilage and bone, causing deformity

Incidence and Demographics
- The incidence of JIA is 1 per 100,000 children
- Girls have a higher incidence than boys
- The peak onset times are 1–3 years of age and 8–10 years of age

Risk Factors
- Risk factors for JIA have not been identified
- Infection, injury, and surgery may precipitate symptom flare-up in diagnosed children

Prevention and Screening
- There is no prevention for JIA
- Screening for iridocyclitis by an ophthalmologist every 3–12 months
- Screening for osteoporosis

Assessment
History
- Morning stiffness
- Fatigue or irritability
- Fever
- Weight loss

Physical Exam
- Joint warmth, swelling, tenderness, loss of mobility
- Growth retardation
- Oligoarticular JIA
  - Fewer than five affected joints
  - Knees and wrists most often affected
  - Can cause iridocyclitis, inflammation of the iris and ciliary body
  - Iridocyclitis may result in cataracts, glaucoma, loss of vision
  - Signs of iridocyclitis include red eyes, diminished vision, unequal pupils, eye pain, and headaches
- Polyarticular JIA
  - Five or more affected joints
  - Hands and feet most often affected

- Systemic JIA
  - Daily high-spiking fevers
  - Intermittent rash
  - Variable joint involvement
  - Hepatosplenomegaly
  - Enlarged lymph nodes

Diagnostic Studies
- No definitive studies for JIA
- Elevated white blood cells during flare-up of symptoms
- Elevated antinuclear antibodies (ANA) are indicative, not diagnostic
- Elevated ANA indicates higher risk for iridocyclitis
- Rheumatoid factor (RF) positive in 10% of children with JIA
- Erythrocyte sedimentation rate (ESR) may or may not be elevated
- Radiographs or MRI to show condition of joints

Management

Invasive Management
- No invasive management indicated

Nonpharmacologic Management
- Physical therapy to maintain muscle tone, improve mobility, prevent joint damage
- Occupational therapy to improve performance of activities of daily living
- Splinting during rest to relieve pain and prevent flexion deformity
- Warm, moist heat
- Relaxation techniques, guided imagery, distraction to cope with discomfort

Pharmacologic Management
- Nonsteroidal anti-inflammatory drugs (NSAIDs)
  - Ibuprofen (Motrin) or Naproxen (Naprosyn)
  - To decrease inflammation, relieve pain, minimize joint damage
- Disease-modifying antirheumatic drugs (DMARDs)
- Methotrexate
  - To prevent bone and joint destruction by suppressing the immune system attack on joints
- Biological immunomodulators
  - Etanercept (Enbrel)
  - To block binding of tumor necrosis factor with cell surface receptors to reduce proinflammatory activity
- Growth hormone to combat growth retardation

Patient/Family Education
- Disease process and treatment plan
- Splint therapy
- Nonpharmacologic management
- Medication administration

Outcomes and Follow-Up
- The child will have maximum mobility.
- The child will remain comfortable with effective pain management.
- The child will complete activities of daily living independently.
- The child will experience minimal symptom flare-ups.
- The child will maintain growth within normal limits.
- The child will be screened regularly by ophthalmologist.
- The child and family will verbalize understanding of disease and treatment plan.
- The child and family will demonstrate splint therapy and strategies for nonpharmacologic management.
- The child and family will demonstrate effective medication administration.

IDIOPATHIC SCOLIOSIS

Description
Idiopathic scoliosis is lateral spinal curvature of more than 10°. The disorder has three categories based on age of initial presentation. Infantile idiopathic scoliosis presents in children before the age of 3 years, the juvenile form between 3 and 10 years, and the adolescent form between 11 and 17 years.

Etiology
The exact cause is unknown, but is considered to be multifactorial.

Incidence and Demographics
- 3%–5% of the population has scoliosis, but less than 1% of those affected require treatment
- Adolescent idiopathic scoliosis is more prevalent in females

Risk Factors
- There are no identified risk factors

Prevention and Screening
- There is no prevention
- Screening was traditionally performed in school, but has become controversial due to high number of unnecessary referrals

Assessment
History
- Progression of physical signs

Physical Exam
- Uneven shoulders, scapula, or waistline
- Tilt of pelvis
- Visible curve

Diagnostic Studies
- Radiography to evaluate degree of curve and skeletal maturity
- MRI scan

Management
Invasive
- Surgical correction for curves greater than 50°
- Fusion of vertebrae
- Internal instrumentation with screw, rods to hold fusion in place

Nonpharmacologic
- Treatment is not necessary if curve is less than 20° and nonprogressive
- External spinal orthotics (braces) for curves greater than or equal to 20°
- Exercises to slow progression
- Postoperative care:
  - Pressure-relieving mattress
  - Long roll to turn depending on specific surgery
  - Foley catheter or chest tube depending on site of repair
  - Progressive ambulation and physical therapy
  - Adequate fluid intake and high fiber foods to prevent constipation

Pharmacologic
- Postoperative pain management
- Postoperative stool softeners to prevent constipation

Patient/Family Education
- Explanation of defect and treatment plan
- Exercise therapy
- Care of external spinal orthotic
- Pain management
- Progressive ambulation

Outcomes and Follow-Up
- The child will have maximum mobility.
- The child's skin will remain intact.
- The child will participate in an exercise plan.
- The child will experience effective postoperative pain management.
- The child will follow plan for progressive ambulation.
- The child and family will verbalize understanding of defect and treatment plan.
- The child and family will demonstrate application and care of external orthotic.

SLIPPED CAPITAL FEMORAL EPIPHYSIS (SCFE)

Description
Slipped capital femoral epiphysis (SCFE) is an acquired disorder of the hip in which the head of the femur separates from the rest of the femur. The condition occurs in preadolescent and adolescent children.

Etiology
- Most cases of SCFE are idiopathic.
- Multifactorial etiology may include local injury, obesity causing pressure on growth plate, inflammatory factors, and endocrinologic factors.
- The pressure on the femoral head exceeds the resistance of the growth plate, causing the neck of the femur to slip anteriorly.

Incidence and Demographics
- Incidence is 2–10 adolescents per 100,000
- Usually occurs at time of growth spurt, with peak occurrence at 10–13 years in females and 12–16 years in males
- Higher incidence in males, Pacific Islanders, and Blacks
- Rare in females after onset of menses
- The incidence of SCFE of the initially unaffected hip is 25%–40% and may occur 6–12 months later

Risk Factors
- Obesity with body mass index (BMI) greater than the 95th percentile
- May be associated with hypothyroidism, growth hormone administration, renal osteodystrophy, previous radiation therapy

Prevention and Screening
- Weight management
- Evaluation of limp and/or pain in hip, thigh, or knee

Assessment
History
- Groin, thigh, or knee pain
- Exacerbation of pain after trauma such as a fall or sports injury

Physical Exam
- Pain in hip, groin, thigh, or knee
- Limp or gait abnormalities
- Limited range of hip motion
- Inability to bear weight with unstable SCFE
- Ability to bear weight with stable SCFE
- External rotation and abduction of hip with flexion
- Mild atrophy of thigh and gluteal muscles with chronic involvement

Diagnostic Studies
- Radiographs to show degree of slippage
- MRI to show bone edema around the growth plate if radiograph appears normal

Management
Invasive Management
- Surgical placement of screw through the femoral neck into the femoral epiphysis
- Radiographic guidance allows for small incision with minimal blood loss

Nonpharmacologic Management
- Crutches or wheelchair
- Partial or no weight-bearing for 6–8 weeks following surgery
- Monitor incision for redness, swelling, or drainage
- Sports restrictions for 3–6 months

Patient/Family Education
- No weight-bearing on affected leg to prevent further slippage
- Wound care and assessment
- Safe ambulation with crutches or wheelchair
- Importance of follow-up visits

Outcomes and Follow-Up
- The child will adhere to mobility restrictions.
- The child's incision site will heal without infection.
- The child will demonstrate safe use of crutches or wheelchair.
- The child will not experience complications such as avascular necrosis of the femoral head, acute cartilage necrosis (chondrolysis), or early onset of degenerative arthritis.
- The child will be monitored for slippage of uninvolved hip.
- The child and family will adhere to follow-up visit schedule.

BONE TUMORS

Description
Osteogenic sarcoma, also known as osteosarcoma, arises from the bone-forming cells. This cancer most commonly occurs in the knee, femur, tibia, and humerus. Metastasis may involve the lung and other bones.

Ewing sarcoma is another primary bone tumor occurring in the bone (osseous) or in the soft tissue (extraosseous). Common sites include femur, fibula, tibia, foot, pelvis, humerus, scapula, radius, ulna, hand, rib, vertebrae, clavicle, mandible, and skull. Metastasis is to lung, bone, and bone marrow.

Etiology
The cause is unknown.

Incidence and Demographics

Osteogenic sarcoma and Ewing sarcoma constitute 85% of all primary malignant bone tumors in children. The peak incidence is 15–19 years of age. Bone neoplasms affect males and females equally until puberty, when males are affected twice as often as females. The 5-year disease-free survival rate for localized osteogenic sarcoma is 75%–80%; with metastases, the rate is 10%–45%. The 5-year disease–free survival rate for localized Ewing sarcoma is 65%–76%; with metastases, the rate drops to 30%.

Risk Factors

- No risk factors have been identified

Prevention and Screening

- There is no prevention
- Evaluation of bone pain, localized swelling, mobility limitations, bone fractures

Assessment

History

- Complaints of fever, weight loss, pain, swelling, limited mobility without associated trauma

Physical Exam

- Localized swelling, mass
- Limited mobility
- Aching pain
- Fracture
- Ewing sarcoma may be accompanied by fever and weight loss

Diagnostic Studies

- Radiographs
- MRI
- CT scan
- Bone scan
- Bone marrow biopsy
- Elevated sedimentation rate may accompany Ewing sarcoma

Management

Invasive

- Surgical resection
- Amputation
- Limb salvage surgery

Nonpharmacologic

- Radiation therapy

Pharmacologic

- Osteogenic sarcoma
  - Methotrexate
  - Doxorubicin (Adriamycin)

- – Cyclophosphamide (Cytoxan)
- – Cisplatin (Platinol)
- – Ifosfamide (Ifos)
- – Etoposide (VP-16, VePesid)
- – Carboplatin (CBDCA)
- Ewing sarcoma
  - – Vincristine (Oncovin)
  - – Doxorubicin (Adriamycin)
  - – Ifosfamide (Ifos)
  - – Etoposide (VP-16, VePesid)
  - – Most protocols include cyclophosphamide (Cytoxan)
  - – Some include dactinomycin (Actinomycin D)

Patient/Family Education
- Preparation for diagnostic procedures
- Side effects of radiation and chemotherapy
- Signs of infection, anemia, low platelet count
- Infection prevention
- Strategies for coping with low platelet count, stomatitis, nausea and vomiting, constipation, decreased appetite, fatigue, alopecia

Outcomes and Follow-Up
- The child will receive prompt treatment for complications of chemotherapy and radiation.
- The child will not experience infection.
- The child will have balanced nutritional intake.
- The child will experience effective pain management.
- The child and family will verbalize understanding of the disease, diagnostic procedures, and treatment.

REFERENCES

Adam, S. P., & Talwalker, V. R. (2007). Legg-Calvé-Perthes disease. *Current Opinion in Orthopaedics, 18, 544–549.*

Berg, E. E. (2006). Osteogenic sarcoma. *Orthopedic Nursing, 25,* 348–349.

Carson, S., Woolridge, D. P., Colletti, J., & Kilgore, K. (2006). Pediatric upper extremity injuries. *Pediatric Clinics of North America, 53,* 41–67.

Dezateux, C., & Rosendahl, K. (2007). Developmental dysplasia of the hip. *Lancet, 369,* 1541–1552.

Faulks, S., & Luther, B. (2005). Changing paradigm for the treatment of clubfeet. *Orthopaedic Nursing, 24,* 25–30.

Goldberg, C. J., Moore, D. P., Fogarty, E. E., & Dowling, F. E. (2008). Scoliosis: a review. *Pediatric Surgery International, 24,* 129–144.

Gore, A. I., & Spencer, J. P. (2004). The newborn foot. *American Family Physician, 69,* 865–872.

Goulding, A. (2007). Risk factors for fractures in normally active children and adolescents. *Medicine and Sports Science, 51,* 102–120.

Guell, C. (2007). Painful childhood: Children living with juvenile arthritis. *Qualitative Health Research, 17,* 884–892.

Hart, E. S., Albright, M. B., Rebello, G. N., & Grottkau, B. E. (2006a). Developmental dysplasia of the hip: nursing implications and anticipatory guidance for parents. *Orthopaedic Nursing, 25,* 100–109.

Hart, E. S., Albright, M. B., Rebello, G. N., & Grottkau, B. E. (2006b). Broken bones: Common pediatric fractures. *Orthopaedic Nursing, 25,* 251–256.

Hart, E. S., Grottkau, B. E., & Albright, M. B. (2007). Slipped capital femoral epiphysis: Don't miss this pediatric hip disorder. *The Nurse Practitioner, 32*(3), 14–21.

Hart, E. S., Grottkau, B. E., Rebello, G. N., & Albright, M. B. (2006). Broken bones: Common pediatric upper extremity fractures. *Orthopaedic Nursing, 25,* 311–323.

Hart, E. S., Luther, B., & Grottkau, B. E. (2006). Broken bones: Common pediatric lower extremity fractures. *Orthopaedic Nursing, 25,* 390–407.

Hockenberry, M. J., & Wilson, D. (2007). *Wong's nursing care of infants and children.* St. Louis, MO: Mosby Elsevier.

Hoffmeister, E. (2008). Research sheds greater light on Legg-Calvé-Perthes disease. *Bone and Joint, 14,* 3–5.

Iwinski, H. J. (2006). Slipped capital femoral epiphysis. *Current Opinion in Orthopaedics, 17,* 511–516.

Junnila, J. L., & Cartwright, V. W. (2006a). Chronic musculoskeletal pain in children: Part I. Initial evaluation. *American Family Physician, 74,* 115–122.

Junnila, J. L., & Cartwright, V. W. (2006b). Chronic musculoskeletal pain in children: Part II. Rheumatic causes. *American Family Physician, 74,* 293–300.

Lahl, M., Fisher, V. L., & Laschinger, K. (2008). Ewing's sarcoma family of tumors: An overview from diagnosis to survivorship. *Clinical Journal of Oncology Nursing, 12,* 89–97.

McCarthy, J. J., Dormans, J. P., Kozin, S. H., & Pezzutillo, P. D. (2004). Musculoskeletal infections in children: Basic treatment principles and recent advancements. *The Journal of Bone & Joint Surgery, 86-A,* 850–863.

Morcuende, J. A., Dolan, L. A., Dietz, F. R., & Ponseti, I. V. (2004). Radical reduction in the rate of extensive corrective surgery for clubfoot using the Ponseti method. *Pediatrics, 113,* 376–380.

North American Spine Society. *Adolescent idiopathic scoliosis.* Retrieved from http://www.spine.org/Pages/ConsumerHealth/SpineConditionsAndTreatments/CommonProblemsCorrectiveActions/OtherConditionsInjuries/Scoliosis,AdolescentIdiopathic.aspx

Schoen, D. C. (2006). Bone neoplasms. *Orthopaedic Nursing, 25,* 427–430.

Shuman, T. (2006). Juvenile rheumatoid arthritis. *WebMD Health.* Retrieved from http://www.medscape.com/viewarticle/490244

Storer, S. K., & Skaggs, D. L. (2006). Developmental dysplasia of the hip. *American Family Physician, 74,* 1310–1316.

Taylor, M. N., Chaudhuri, R., Davis, J., Novelli, V., & Jaswon, M. S. (2007). Childhood osteomyelitis presenting as a pathological fracture. *Clinical Radiology, 63,* 348–351.

U.S. Preventative Services Task Force. (2006). *Screening for developmental dysplasia of the hip: recommendation statement.* Retrieved from http://www.ahrq.gov/clinic/uspstf06/hipdysp/hipdysrs.htm

Integumentary Disorders

Clara J. Richardson, MSN, RN-BC

ECZEMA

Description
Eczema, or atopic dermatitis, is a chronic inflammatory skin disorder.

Etiology
Exacerbation of eczema may be triggered by exposure to skin irritants such as soaps and laundry detergents, skin infections, food, or inhaled allergens.

Incidence and Demographics
Eczema affects 5%–7% of children and the peak incidence is between 6 months and 8–10 years of age. About 95% of children with eczema have asthma or allergic rhinitis.

Risk Factors
- Family history

Prevention and Screening
- No prevention or screening indicated

Assessment

History
- Dry skin
- Asthma or allergic rhinitis

Physical Exam
- Skin redness, dryness
- Itching
- Irritability
- Vesicles or papules with weeping, crusting
- Lichenification, thickened skin areas

Diagnostic Studies
- No diagnostic studies indicated

Management

Invasive
- No invasive management indicated

Nonpharmacologic
- Daily lubrication with emollient such as Eucerin, Aquaphor, Cetaphil
- Tepid bath with mild skin cleaner or colloidal bath product
- Cool, wet compresses
- Hypoallergenic diet for identified food allergies
- Keep fingernails and toenails short
- Gloves or socks to prevent scratching
- Soft, cotton clothing and bedding
- Avoid overheating
- Mild laundry detergent without fabric softener

Pharmacologic
- Topical steroid for short periods
- Topical immunomodulators:
  - Tacrolimus (Protopic)
  - Pimecrolimus (Elidel)
- Antihistamine for itching:
  - Diphenhydramine (Benadryl)
  - Hydroxyzine (Atarax)
- Antibiotics for secondary bacterial infection

Patient/Family Education
- Diagnosis and treatment plan
- Daily skin care
- Care during exacerbations
- Medication administration
- Signs of bacterial infection: worsening of lesions, fever, malaise

Outcomes and Follow-Up
- The child will maintain intact skin.
- The child will show evidence of healing skin.
- The child will demonstrate relief from itching.
- The child will not develop secondary bacterial infection.
- The family will verbalize understanding of diagnosis and treatment plan.
- The family will identify triggers of exacerbation.
- The family will demonstrate effective daily skin care and care during exacerbations.
- The family will demonstrate medication administration.
- The family will recognize signs of bacterial infection.

IMPETIGO

Description
Impetigo is a highly contagious bacterial infection of the skin.

Etiology
Staphylococcus aureus is the most common cause, with fewer cases from *Streptococcus pyogenes*. The organism affects the superficial epidermis layer of the skin and may be a primary or secondary infection. Impetigo may be spread by direct contact or indirectly by contact with clothing or toys.

Incidence and Demographics
Impetigo may occur at any age, but is most prevalent in children 2–5 years of age. The nonbullous form of impetigo accounts for approximately 70% of cases. The bullous form can occur at any age, but is most prevalent in newborns. The most common sites for the nonbullous form are face and limbs; for the bullous form, the most common sites are neck folds, nose, groin, and axillae.

Risk Factors
- Renal dialysis
- Immune deficiency disorders
- Poor hygiene
- Crowded living conditions

Prevention and Screening
- Prevention consists of avoiding exposure
- No screening indicated

Assessment
History
- Insect bites
- Varicella

Physical Exam
- Nonbullous form: Small vesicles or pustules that rupture, with honey-colored crusty exudate
- Bullous form: Blisters that rupture easily, leaving erythematous lesions
- Itching

Diagnostic Studies
- Culture of lesion

Management
Invasive
- No invasive management indicated

Nonpharmacologic
- Meticulous handwashing
- Daily bath, clothing change
- Wash clothing, bedding in hot water
- Wash toys and avoid sharing with unaffected children
- Contact infection control precautions

Pharmacologic
- Topical antibiotics:
  - Retapamulin (Altabax)
  - Mupirocin (Bactroban)
- Oral antibiotics for extensive disease:
  - Amoxicillin/clavulanate (Augmentin)
  - Cefuroxime (Ceftin)
  - Cephalexin (Keflex)

Patient/Family Education
- Diagnosis and treatment plan
- Medication administration
- Strategies to prevent spread of infection

Outcomes and Follow-Up
- The child will regain clear, intact skin.
- The child will experience relief of itching.
- The child will not spread infection to others.
- The family will verbalize understanding of diagnosis and treatment plan.
- The family will demonstrate medication administration.
- The family will identify strategies to prevent spread of infection.

CELLULITIS

Description
Cellulitis is an acute bacterial infection of the skin and subcutaneous tissue.

Etiology
Common causative organisms are Group A beta-hemolytic streptococci and *Staphylococcus aureus*, including methicillin-resistant S. aureus (MRSA). Areas most affected are face, lower extremities, periorbital, and perianal.

Incidence and Demographics
- Incidence is approximately 2–3 cases per 100 people each year

Risk Factors
- Trauma or surgery
- Peripheral vascular disease
- Diabetes
- Overcrowded living conditions

Prevention and Screening
- No prevention or screening indicated

Assessment
History
- Fever
- Malaise
- History of trauma or surgery

Physical Exam
- Erythema
- Edema
- Pain
- Hot and tender to touch
- Red streaking of surrounding skin
- Diagnostic studies
- Complete blood count
- Blood cultures
- CT scan to rule out abscess, a complication
- Culture of abscess

Management
Invasive
- No invasive management for simple cellulitis
- Incision and drainage may be necessary for abscess

Nonpharmacologic
- Elevate affected extremity
- Warm compress
- Dressing to cover open areas
- Contact infection control precautions

Pharmacologic
- Oral cephalexin (Keflex), clindamycin (Cleocin), amoxicillin-clavulanic acid (Augmentin), or co-trimoxazole (Septra)
- IV clindamycin or vancomycin
- Analgesics for pain

Patient/Family Education
- Disease process and treatment plan
- Strategies to prevent spread of infection
- Nonpharmacologic management
- Medication administration

Outcomes and Follow-Up
- The child's skin integrity is maintained with decrease in symptoms.
- The child will experience effective pain management.
- The child will not experience abscess formation.
- The family will verbalize understanding of disease process and treatment plan.
- The family will identify strategies to prevent spread of infection.
- The family will utilize nonpharmacologic management.
- The family will demonstrate effective pain management.

COMMUNICABLE DISEASES

Description
Communicable diseases with skin manifestations are illnesses caused by infectious agents.

Etiology

Exanthema Subitum (Roseola)
- Human herpesvirus type 6 (HHV-6) transmitted through respiratory secretions
- Incubation period 5–15 days
- Complications
  - Febrile seizures
  - Rare occurrence of complications

Erythema Infectiosum (Fifth Disease)
- Human parvovirus B19 (PV-B19) transmitted through respiratory droplets, blood products, mother to fetus
- Incubation period 4–14 days
- Complications:
  - Aplastic crisis
  - Congenital infection

Rubeola (Measles)
- Highly contagious virus transmitted through respiratory droplets
- Incubation period 10–20 days
- Complications most common with children younger than 5 years and adults
    - Respiratory: Otitis media, laryngotracheobronchitis, pneumonia
    - Neurological: Febrile seizures, encephalitis
    - Gastrointestinal: Diarrhea
    - Ophthalmic: Inflammation of cornea, blindness
    - Hematologic: Thrombocytopenic purpura, disseminated intravascular coagulation
    - Cardiovascular: Myocarditis, pericarditis
    - Cellulitis, nephritis

Rubella (German measles, 3-day measles)
- Virus transmitted through respiratory droplets, mother to fetus
- Incubation period 14–21 days
- Complications:
    - Congenital deafness, eye abnormalities, congenital heart disease, cognitive impairment, fetal death
    - Rarely: Arthritis, encephalitis, thrombocytopenic purpura, hepatitis

Varicella (Chickenpox)
- Varicella-zoster virus transmitted by respiratory droplets, contact with lesions, mother to fetus
- Incubation period 14–16 days
- Complications rare
    - Secondary infection
    - Varicella encephalitis
    - Varicella pneumonia

Incidence and Demographics
Exanthema Subitum (Roseola)
- 12%–30% incidence
- 86% of children have HHV-6 antibodies by age 1
- Peak occurrence in spring and fall

Erythema Infectiosum (Fifth Disease)
- Most common at 3–15 years of age
- Peak occurrence in late winter or early spring

Rubeola (Measles)
- 0.02 per 100,000 people
- 55 cases in 2006
- More common during the winter among the unimmunized

Rubella (German Measles)
- No longer endemic in the United States
- 11 cases in 2006
- More common in winter and spring

Varicella (Chickenpox)
- 28.65 per 100,000 people
- Most cases occur in winter and early spring

Risk Factors
- Exposure to causative agent
- Immunocompromised state

Prevention and Screening
- Exanthema subitum (roseola): No prevention or screening
- Erythema infectiosum (fifth disease): No prevention or screening
- Rubeola (measles)
  - Measles, mumps, and rubella vaccine (MMR)
  - First dose at 12–18 months of age and second at 4–6 years
  - Screen adolescents and young adults for susceptibility
  - Postexposure vaccine within 72 hours
  - Postexposure Ig within 6 days for pregnant women
- Rubella (German measles): See MMR
  - Screen women of childbearing age for susceptibility
  - Immunize unless pregnant
  - Postexposure Ig, but not in pregnant women
- Varicella (chickenpox)
  - Varicella vaccine
  - First dose at 12–18 months of age and second at 4–6 years
  - Postexposure varicella-zoster immune globulin (VZIG) for susceptible individuals

Assessment
History
- Exanthema subitum (roseola): Fever for about 3 days, decreased temperature, rash appearance
- Erythema infectiosum (fifth disease): Very mild with headache, low-grade fever, sore throat, malaise, nausea
- Rubeola (measles): Fever, cough, conjunctivitis, Koplik spots (small, red, raised spots with whitish-bluish center on buccal mucosa)
- Rubella (German measles): Eye pain, conjunctivitis, sore throat, headache, low-grade fever, nausea, body aches
- Varicella (chickenpox): Low-grade fever, malaise, anorexia, headache, sore throat

Physical Exam
EXANTHEMA SUBITUM (ROSEOLA)
- Faint red, maculopapular, nonitching rash mainly on trunk that fades on pressure and lasts for a few hours to a few days
- Erythematous papules on soft palate and uvula
- Fever
- Cough
- Diarrhea

ERYTHEMA INFECTIOSUM (FIFTH DISEASE)
- First stage: Bright red, nonitching rash over cheeks lasting 2–4 days
- Second stage: Red maculopapular, nonitching rash on extremities appearing about 1 day after first stage and lasting about a week
- Third stage: Second stage rash fades into lacy pattern, appearing off and on for up to 3 weeks

RUBEOLA (MEASLES)
- Progressive rash with discrete, red, maculopapular spots
- Photophobia
- Sore throat
- Headache
- Abdominal pain
- Swollen lymph nodes

RUBELLA (GERMAN MEASLES)
- Progressive, pinkish-red, discrete, maculopapular rash
- Fever
- Swollen lymph nodes
- Petechiae on soft palate

VARICELLA (CHICKENPOX)
- Itchy, red, papular rash becomes vesicular and then breaks, forming crusts by day 7
- Rash may spread to mouth, conjunctivae, genital area

Diagnostic Studies
- Diagnosis based on symptoms

Management
Invasive
- No invasive management indicated

Nonpharmacologic
- Rest
- Extra fluids
- Low lighting for measles
- Mittens at night to prevent scratching with chickenpox
- Isolate from susceptible individuals
- Droplet infection control precautions
- Airborne infection control precautions for rubeola (measles)
- Airborne and contact infection control precautions for varicella (chickenpox)

Pharmacologic
- Acetaminophen (Tylenol) or ibuprofen (Motrin) for fever or discomfort
- Antihistamine (Benadryl) for itching

Patient/Family Education
- Disease process
- Prevention of transmission
- Comfort measures
- Medication administration

Outcomes and Follow-Up
- The child will experience relief from fever, discomfort, and itching.
- The child will not experience complications.
- The child will maintain skin integrity.
- The family will verbalize understanding of disease.
- The family will utilize strategies to prevent spread of infection.
- The family will demonstrate comfort measures and medication administration.

FUNGAL INFECTIONS

Description
Fungal infections are superficial skin infections caused by dermatophytes, a group of fungi. The three most common fungal infections affecting children are tinea capitis (ringworm of the scalp), tinea corporis (ringworm of the skin), and candidiasis (moniliasis), which grows in warm, moist areas of the body.

Etiology
- Tinea capitis: *Trichophyton tonsurans*, *Microsporum audouinii*, *Microsporum canis*
- Tinea corporis: *Trichophyton rubrum*, *Trichophyton mentagrophytes*, *M. canis*, and *Epidermophyton*
- Candidiasis: *Candida albicans*

Incidence and Demographics
Tinea Capitis
- More prevalent in Blacks and Hispanics
- *M. canis* more prevalent in males
- Peak incidence in children between 1 and 10 years of age

Tinea Corporis
- Peak incidence in preadolescents
- May be carried by household pets

Candidiasis
- Invasive candidiasis is the most common invasive fungal infection in the United States

Risk Factors
- Tendency toward other allergic reactions (tinea capitis and corporis)
- Altered immune status (candidiasis)
- Antibiotic therapy (candidiasis)

Prevention and Screening
- Screening of others in household, classroom, or daycare
- Treatment of asymptomatic family members with medication and shampoo
- Avoid sharing hair brushes, towels, clothing
- Mouth care and diaper care

Assessment
History
- Exposure

Physical Exam
TINEA CAPITIS
- Hair loss and breaking
- Erythema
- Scaling and itching
- Oval patches
- Pustules
- Kerion formation indicates secondary infection: lesions are spongy, raised, with pus drainage
- Scarring if kerion not treated

TINEA CORPORIS
- Round or oval patch
- Erythema
- Scaling

CANDIDIASIS MAY MANIFEST AS ORAL LESIONS (THRUSH) OR AS DIAPER DERMATITIS
- Erythema
- White exudates
- Peeling and bleeding
- Itching
- Pain

Diagnostic Studies
- KOH (potassium hydroxide) microscopic examination
- Wood's ultraviolet lamp
- Culture

Management
Invasive
- No invasive management indicated

Nonpharmacologic
TINEA CAPITIS
- Shampoos to decrease scaling and itching: 2% ketoconazole, 1%–2.5% selenium sulfide, 1%–2% zinc pyrithione, and povidone-iodine
- Cleaning environment
- Personal hygiene

TINEA CORPORIS
- Cleaning environment
- Personal hygiene

CANDIDIASIS
- Mouth care
- Strategies to prevent diaper dermatitis

Pharmacologic
TINEA CAPITIS: ORAL ANTIFUNGALS
- Griseofulvin (Fulvicin)
- Itraconazole (Sporanox)
- Fluconazole (Diflucan)
- Prednisolone (Orapred) for kerions

TINEA CORPORIS: TOPICAL ANTIFUNGALS
- Miconazole (Mycostatin)
- Clotrimazole (Lotrimin)
- Terbinafine (Lamisil)

CANDIDIASIS: TOPICAL ANTIFUNGALS
- Nystatin (Mycostatin)
- Miconazole (Monistat)
- Clotrimazole (Lotrimin)

Patient/Family Education
- Disease process and treatment plan
- Prevention of spread of infection
- Nonpharmacologic management
- Medication administration

Outcomes and Follow-Up
- The child will recover with intact, lesion-free skin.
- The family will verbalize understanding of disease and treatment plan.
- The family will demonstrate medication administration.
- The family will identify strategies to prevent spread of infection.
- The family will demonstrate nonpharmacologic management.

PARASITIC INFESTATIONS

Description
Two common parasitic skin infestations in children are scabies and head lice.

Etiology
Scabies is caused by a mite called Sarcoptes scabiei that burrows under the skin, leaving a trail of eggs and feces. Symptoms are due to a hypersensitivity reaction to the feces. Usual sites of infestation in children are finger webs, wrists, axillae, elbows, and buttocks.

Pediculus humanus capitis is caused by parasitic insects commonly called head lice. The female lays eggs at the base of the hair shaft. The eggs hatch in 8–10 days and the nymph feeds on blood. Usual sites are behind the ears and near the neck.

Incidence and Demographics
Head lice occur most often in children age 3–11 and their families. Black children rarely get head lice.

Risk Factors
Scabies
- Skin-to-skin contact
- Crowded living conditions
- Immunocompromised state

Head Lice
- Head-to-head contact
- Less commonly from shared head-contact items such as hats and brushes

Prevention and Screening
Scabies
- Treat household contacts
- Wash contaminated bedding and clothing in hot water and dryer

Head Lice
- Treat household contacts
- Wash contaminated bedding and clothing in hot water and dryer
- Store items that cannot be washed in sealed plastic bag for 2 weeks
- Soak combs and brushes for one hour in alcohol or wash in hot water
- Recheck every few days for 2–3 weeks after infestation
- Avoid sharing of hair gear

Assessment
- History
- History of symptoms

Physical Exam
SCABIES
- Pruritus, especially intense at night
- Burrow looks like a short, wavy line
- Papules are small and red, changing to vesicles and pustules
- Scratching leads to secondary infection
- Crusted appearance indicates hyperinfestation

HEAD LICE
- Pruritus
- Sensation of something moving
- Secondary lesions from scratching

Diagnostic Studies
SCABIES
- Microscopic examination of skin scrapings

HEAD LICE
- Presence of nits on inspection

Management
Invasive
- No invasive management indicated

Nonpharmacologic
SCABIES
- Cool baths to relieve itching
- Avoid scratching, which can lead to secondary bacterial infection
- Wash contaminated bedding and clothing in hot water and dryer
- Contact infection control precautions for first 24 hours after treatment

HEAD LICE
- Wash clothing and bedding used within the last two days
- Avoid rewashing hair for at least one day after treatment
- Remove all nits with nit comb
- Contact infection control precautions for first 4 hours after treatment

Pharmacologic

SCABIES
- Permethrin 5% (Elimite) topical solution in single overnight application
- Ivermectin (Stromectol) orally if permethrin not tolerated

HEAD LICE
- Pyrethrins (A-200, Pronto, Rid)
- Permethrin (Nix)
- Malathion (Ovide)

Patient/Family Education
- Diagnosis and treatment plan
- Medication administration
- Strategies to prevent spread

Outcomes and Follow-Up
- The child will be parasite-free after treatment.
- The child will maintain intact skin with no secondary infection.
- The family will verbalize understanding of diagnosis and treatment plan.
- The family will demonstrate medication administration.
- The family will identify strategies to prevent spread of infestation.

ACNE VULGARIS

Description
Acne is an inflammatory skin condition characterized by obstruction of sebaceous follicles.

Etiology
Excessive sebum and desquamated epithelial cells clog pores, *Propionibacterium acnes* proliferates and causes an inflammatory reaction.

Incidence and Demographics
Acne affects 80% of adolescents between the ages of 13 and 18 years.

Risk Factors
- Cosmetics containing lanolin, petrolatum, lauryl alcohol, butyl stearate, and oleic acid
- Exposure to cooking oil with work over fast-food grill

Prevention and Screening
- Avoidance of risk factors may help prevent acne

Assessment

History
• Presence of acne

Physical Exam
• Noninflammatory open comedones, called blackheads
• Noninflammatory closed comedones, called whiteheads
• Reddened papules, pustules, nodules, or cysts
• Scarring may appear as ice-pick marks or more hypertrophic

Diagnostic Studies
• No diagnostic studies indicated

Management

Invasive
• No invasive management indicated

Nonpharmacologic
• Nonabrasive skin cleanser
• Handwashing
• Avoid squeezing or picking, which increases scarring
• Keeping hair shampooed and away from face

Pharmacologic
• Topical antibiotics:
    – Erythromycin: Antibacterial
    – Clindamycin (Cleocin): Antibacterial
    – Benzoyl peroxide with erythromycin or clindamycin: Antibacterial
    – Azelaic acid: Antibacterial, anticomedonal, anti-inflammatory
    – Metronidazole (Metro gel)
• Topical retinoids to loosen comedones, anti-inflammatory:
    – Tretinoin (Retin-A)
    – Adapalene
    – Tazarotene
• Systemic antibiotics:
    – Tetracycline or lymecycline (second generation tetracycline)
    – Erythromycin or azithromycin (derivative of erythromycin)
    – Doxycycline (Vibramycin)
    – Minocycline (Minocin)
    – Trimethoprim-sulfamethoxazole
    – Clindamycin
• Isotretinoin (Accutane) taken orally to decrease sebum
• Hormonal treatment with oral contraceptive pill to decrease sebum

Patient/Family Education
• Disease process
• Treatment options
• Skin care

Outcomes and Follow-Up
- The child will have a decrease in lesions and heal without scarring.
- The child will demonstrate effective skin care.
- The child and family will discuss treatment options and agree on plan of care.

BURNS

Description
A burn is tissue injury due to contact with heat, extreme cold, chemicals, electricity, or radiation.

Etiology
Thermal injuries are due to scalds, hot objects, and flame. Children sustain electrical burns from inserting conductive objects into outlets or chewing on electrical cords. Chemicals may be spilled on skin, splashed in eyes, or ingested. Burn injuries from radiation or extreme cold are rare in children. The body's response to a burn is local or systemic, depending on the severity of the injury.

Local response involves:
- Vasodilation causes increased hydrostatic pressure in the vessels which, coupled with increased capillary permeability, moves fluid into the interstitial spaces, causing edema
- Fluid lost from the burn wound
- Fluid shifts, decreased cardiac output, and edema lead to capillary stasis with tissue ischemia

Systemic response is characterized by:
- Significant decrease in cardiac output and fluid loss, resulting in burn shock
- Fluid shift to interstitial spaces can compress the vessels, causing compartment syndrome
- Reduced renal blood flow can cause acute renal failure
- Ischemia of the gastrointestinal tract can cause necrosis
- Gastric acid production is decreased for up to 3 days, but then accelerates rapidly and can lead to ulceration
- Increased cortisol and catecholamines initiate hypermetabolism that may cause rapid protein breakdown, lipid catabolism, and muscle wasting
- Anemia and metabolic acidosis occur
- Production of growth hormone diminishes and growth is delayed

Incidence and Demographics
Burn injury is the fifth leading cause of nonfatal, unintentional injury in U.S. children under 1 year of age; the eighth in 1–4-year-olds. The incidence of burn injury is 166.9/100,000 children between ages 0–19. These injuries account for 0.65 deaths/100,000 in this age group.

Risk Factors
- Young children are more likely to sustain burn injury
- Use of heating devices such as kerosene heaters and wood-burning stoves
- Inadequate supervision by adults
- Lack of home safety precautions

Prevention and Screening
There is no screening, but many ways to prevent burns in children

Kitchen Safety
- Stove guards; pot handles and hot liquids out of reach
- Avoid tablecloths and drinking hot liquids with child on lap
- Keep child out of kitchen during food preparation

Bath Safety
- Lower temperature of water heaters to 120°F
- Constant supervision of young children

Home Safety
- Keep matches, lighters, candles, flammables out of reach
- Keep electrical cords out of reach, use outlet covers
- Working smoke detectors, emergency escape plan
- Flame-retardant sleepwear

Outside Safety
- No fireworks for children
- Keep children away from grills, fire pits
- Sun protection

Assessment
History
- Details of burn injury

Physical Exam
- Extent of injury: total body surface area (TBSA) burned
- Depth of injury

SEVERITY OF INJURY
- Minor: < 10% TBSA, partial thickness
- Moderate: 10%–20% TBSA, partial thickness
- Major: > 20% TBSA, all full thickness

Table 18-1. Types of Burns

1st degree	Superficial	Red, pain of epidermis only
2nd degree	Partial thickness	Blisters, pain, swelling of epidermis and dermis
3rd degree	Full thickness	White, brown, charred, blisters, little or no pain
4th degree	Full thickness	Involves skin, muscle, and bone

INHALATION INJURY
- Facial or neck edema
- Singed nasal hairs
- Hoarseness
- Difficulty breathing
- Stridor, wheezing, rales
- Restricted chest movement due to encircling burn

Diagnostic Studies
- Arterial blood gases
- Chest radiography
- Complete blood counts
- Type and crossmatch
- Coagulation studies
- Chemistry panel
- Electrocardiogram (ECG)

Management

Invasive
- Escharotomy, incision of burned tissue, to relieve compartment syndrome
- Excision and debridement
- Skin grafts provide permanent coverage
- Cultured epithelium grown from the child's skin

Nonpharmacologic
- Intubation and artificial ventilation for >20% TBSA or inhalation injury
- 100% humidified oxygen to relieve carbon monoxide poisoning
- Nasogastric tube for decompression
- Early high-protein, high-carbohydrate enteral feeding
- Increase environmental temperature to 31.5° C (88.7° F)
- Foley catheter to monitor urine output
- Cool compresses only for <10% TBSA burned
- Hydrotherapy
- Wash chemical burns with water for 20 minutes
- Progressive dressing changes
- Temporary skin substitutes to promote healing:
  - Allograft (homograft) cadaver skin lasts about 14 days
  - Porcine xenograft lasts 2–3 days
  - Synthetic skin coverings for partial thickness burns
  - Artificial skin (Integra) for partial or full thickness burns
- Standard infection control precautions including gown, gloves, cap, and mask

Pharmacologic
- Fluid resuscitation to maintain urine output of 0.5–2 ml/kg/hr
- Intravenous albumin after 18–24 hours to maintain serum level
- Topical antimicrobials:
  - Silver sulfadiazine (Silvadene)
  - Mafenide (Sulfamylon)
  - Bacitracin for small areas of minor burn
- Histamine-2 (H2) blockers and/or antacids to prevent stress ulcer
- Ophthalmic ointment for eye abrasions
- Tetanus immunoprophylaxis
- Pain management

Patient/Family Education
- Extent and implications of burn injury
- Treatment plan
- Pain management
- Prevention of future injury

Outcomes and Follow-Up
- The child will maintain open airway and effective circulation.
- The child will maintain body temperature between 98.6° and 100.5° F (37°–38° C).
- The child will maintain fluid and electrolyte balance.
- The child will show evidence of wound healing.
- The child will receive adequate nutrition.
- The child will attain optimal mobility.
- The child will experience effective pain management.
- The child will not experience complications such as pneumonia, respiratory failure, wound infection, septicemia.
- The family will verbalize understanding of burn injury and treatment plan.
- The family will demonstrate effective pain management including medications and nonpharmacological interventions to help child cope with pain.
- The family will monitor skin grafts for signs of infection and bleeding.
- The family will utilize prevention strategies to prevent future injury.

REFERENCES

American Burn Association. (2007). *National burn repository 2007 report.* Retrieved from http://www.ameriburn.org/2007NBRAnnualReport/Report.pdf

Banatvala, J. E., & Brown, D. W. G. (2004). Rubella. *Lancet, 363,* 1127–1137.

Carpenter Rose, E. A., & Hedayati, T. (2007). *Candidiasis.* Retrieved from http://www.emedicine.com/emerg/topic76.htm

Centers for Disease Control and Prevention. (2005). *Treating head lice.* Retrieved from http://www.cdc.gov/ncidod/dpd/parasites/lice/2005_PDF_Treating_Head_Lice.pdf

Centers for Disease Control and Prevention. (2006). *Summary of notifiable diseases—United States, 2006.* Retrieved from http://www.cdc.gov/mmwr/PDF/wk/mm5553.pdf

Centers for Disease Control and Prevention. (2008). *Head lice infestation.* Retrieved from http://www.cdc.gov/ncidod/dpd/parasites/lice/factsht_head_lice.htm

Cole, C., & Gazewood, J. (2007). Diagnosis and treatment of impetigo. *American Family Physician, 75,* 859–864.

Curtis, D. L. (2007). *Cellulitis.* Retrieved from http:www.emedicine.com/emerg/topic88.htm

Drago, D. A. (2005). Kitchen scalds and thermal burns in children five years and younger. *Pediatrics, 115,* 10–16.

Edwards, M. (2008). Prescribing for acne. *Practice Nurse, 35*(2), 26–29.

Hammig, B. J., & Ogletree, R. J. (2006). Burn injuries among infants and toddlers in the United States, 1997–2002. *American Journal of Health Behavior, 30,* 259–267.

Hennemann, S., Crawford, P., & Nguyen, L. (2007). What is the best initial treatment for orbital cellulitis in children? *The Journal of Family Practice, 56,* 662–664.

Heukelbach, J., & Feldmeier, H. (2006), Scabies. *Lancet, 367,* 1767–1774.

Hill, M. J. (2007). Bacterial infections. *Dermatology Nursing, 19,* 562, 572.

Hockenberry, M. J., & Wilson, D. (2007). *Wong's nursing care of infants and children.* St. Louis, MO: Mosby Elsevier.

Katsambas, A., & Dessinioti, C. (2008). New and emerging treatments in dermatology: Acne. *Dermatologic Therapy, 21,* 86–95.

Khangura, S., Wallace, J., Kissoon, N., & Kodeeswaran, T. (2007). Management of cellulitis in a pediatric emergency department. *Pediatric Emergency Care, 23,* 805–811.

Laustsen, G., Shaul, M., & Short, G. (2008). Retapamulin (Altabax). *Nurse Practitioner, 33*(2), 15.

Lewis, L. S. (2007). *Pediatrics, roseola infantum.* Retrieved from http://www.emedicine.com/emerg/topic400.htm

National Collaborating Centre for Women's and Children's Health. (2007). *Atopic eczema in children.* Retrieved from http://www.nice.org.uk/nicemedia/pdf/CG057FullGuideline.pdf

Norbury, W. B., Herndon, D. N., Branski, L. K., Chinkes, D. L., & Jeschke, M. G. (2008). Urinary cortisol and catecholamine excretion after burn injury in children. *Journal of Clinical Endocrinology & Metabolism, 93,* 1270–1275.

Page, T. L., Eiff, M. P., & Judkins, D. Z. (2007). When should you treat scabies empirically. *The Journal of Family Practice, 56,* 570–572.

Perry, R. T., & Halsey, N. A. (2004). The clinical significance of measles: A review. *Journal of Infectious Diseases, 189* (Supplement 1), S4–S16.

Pomerance, H. H. (2005). The usual childhood diseases: Forgotten but not gone. *Fetal and Pediatric Pathology, 24,* 169–189.

Robertson, J., & Shilkofski, N. (Eds.). (2005). *The Harriet Lane handbook.* Philadelphia: Mosby.

Rushing, M. E., Zember, G., & Lesher, J. L. (2006). *Tinea corporis*. Retrieved from http://www.emedicine.com/derm/topic421.htm

Sarabi, K., & Khachemoune, A. (2007). Tinea capitis: A review. *Dermatology Nursing, 19*, 525–529.

Servey, J. T., Reamy, B. V., & Hodge, J. (2007). Clinical presentations of parvovirus B19 infection. *American Family Physician, 75*, 373–376.

Siegel, J. D., Jackson, M., & Chiarello, L. (2007). *2007 guideline for isolation precautions: Preventing transmission of infectious agents in healthcare settings*. Retrieved from http://www.cdc.gov/ncidod/dhqp/pdf/guidelines/Isolation2007.pdf

Silverberg, N., & Block, S. (2008). Uncomplicated skin and skin structure infections in children: Diagnosis and current treatment options in the United States. *Clinical Pediatrics, 47*, 211–219.

Snow, M. (2007). The truth about scabies. *Nursing 2007, 37*(2), 28–30.

Web-based Injury Statistics Query and Reporting System. (2006). *10 leading causes of nonfatal unintentional injury, United States 2006*. Retrieved from http://www.cdc.gov/ncipc.wisquars/nonfatal/quickpicks/quickpicks_2006/unintall.htm

Yaffe, S. J., & Aranda, J. V. (2005). *Neonatal and pediatric pharmacology: Therapeutic principles in practice*. Philadelphia: Lippincott Williams & Wilkins.

Zellman, G. L. (2007). *Erythema infectiosum (fifth disease)*. Retrieved from http://www.emedicine.com/derm/topic136.htm

19

Mental Health Issues in the Child: Acute and Chronic

Paula K. Yim Chiplis, PhD, RN, CPNP, and Mary Jo Gilmer, PhD, MBA, CNS, CNL

AUTISM

Description
Autism is a group of developmental disabilities defined by significant impairments in social interaction and communication skills, usually evident before 3 years of age.

Etiology
Many theories are under study, but no definitive cause has been identified. Typically viewed as a behavioral disorder resulting from abnormal brain function.

Incidence and Demographics
~1 in 500 children, with males 4x more than females

Risk Factors
More common among siblings than in general population. Puberty has been identified as a crucial stage for either showing improvement or deterioration.

Prevention and Screening
- None

Assessment
- Impaired in three domains: Communication, social interaction, and repetitive behaviors
- Withdraws from reality
- Appears indifferent or aversive to affection or physical contact
- May develop seizure disorders or schizophrenia
- Interference with intellect may result in appearance of being mentally retarded
- Lack of meaningful relationships
- Apathy
- Looseness of associations
- Unpredictable, uncontrolled behavior
- May refuse to eat

Management
- Psychotherapy focused on developmental level of child
- Medications: stimulants, neuroleptics, lithium

Outcomes and Follow-Up
- Provide consistent routine in familiar environment
- Set consistent limits
- Prevent self-destructive behavior
- Encourage verbalization
- Physical contact on a regular basis
- Referrals to community resources

FAILURE TO THRIVE (FTT)

Description
Growth failure, commonly used when weight or height falls below the 5th percentile for child's age, or weight curve loss that crosses >2 percentile lines on National Center for Health Statistics growth chart.

Etiology
Cause is often classified as organic (resulting from a physiological condition, such as congenital health defects, neurologic lesions, malabsorption syndrome, chronic infections, gastroesophageal reflux, endocrine dysfunction, or cystic fibrosis). Nonorganic FTT is related to psychosocial factors such as poverty, health beliefs, lack of emotional and sensory stimulation, family stress (parental depression, substance abuse, acute grief).

Incidence and Demographics
Approximately 5% of infants/children are below the 5th percentile for height or weight and may be diagnosed at FTT. Nonorganic causes are more common than organic FTT.

Risk Factors
- An infant/child with physical and/or psychosocial condition as described

Prevention and Screening
- None

Assessment
- Failure to meet developmental milestones, withdrawn, eating disorders, avoidance of eye-to-eye contact, stiff or unyielding body posture

Management
- Treat physical cause of FTT through surgery or medications; assist families with relational issues

Outcomes and Follow-Up
- Focus on supervision and feeding advice rather than repeated measurements that imply poor parenting
- May involve a multidisciplinary healthcare team, behavior modification, and hospitalization
- Consistent caregiver, provision of optimum nutrients, positive feeding environment
- Provide emotional support to parent, confidence-building with parent

DEVELOPMENTAL DISABILITY

Description
A mental or physical disability that is evident before the age of 22 years and likely to continue indefinitely

Etiology
- Learning disability, which is frequently found in association with medical conditions such as lead poisoning, fragile X syndrome, fetal alcohol syndrome
- Impaired motor skills with no definitive cause but may be a response to a chronic illness

Incidence and Demographics
- The national prevalence rate for developmental disabilities in the United States is 1.8%, as established by Gollay and Associates

Risk Factors
- Increased risk for abuse and 4 times more likely to be victims of crime

Prevention and Screening
- None

Assessment
- Difficulty with fluidity and flexibility of thinking
- Dislike of ambiguity (black-and-white thinkers)
- Tendency to concentrate on one aspect of a situation while neglecting others
- Difficulty prioritizing and breaking down tasks into manageable projects
- Tendency to have highly focused areas of expertise and interests
- Tendency for poor generalization skill
- Communication and social problems:
  - Idiosyncratic speech
  - Inability to perceive social cues
  - Difficulty utilizing or understanding nonverbal communication
  - Frequent miscommunications and misunderstandings
  - Tendency toward one-sided conversations
  - Tendency to ask many questions, especially when uncomfortable
  - Tendency to return to familiar, rote questions or subjects of personal interest when anxious
  - Intrusive behavior
  - Poor understanding of the impact of behavior on others
  - Difficulty making and keeping friends

Management
- Slow down speech
- Use visuals whenever possible to reinforce your verbal messages
- Draw pictures
- Write down suggestions for change in brief, outline form
- Present information one item at a time
- Ask for feedback after each item to ensure clear comprehension
- Be specific in making suggestions for change
- Practice different ways of handling tough situations the client is likely to encounter
- Work on building coping skills rather than insight

Outcomes and Follow-Up
- Include a variety of support and education services for families and caregivers

ENURESIS

Description
Involuntary or intentional micturition in inappropriate places, including clothing

Etiology
Contributing factors include slower rate of physical development, positive family history, lengthy duration of sleep in infancy. Primarily an alteration of neuromuscular bladder functioning and generally benign and self-limiting.

Incidence and Demographics
- Types:
  - Primary (enuresis in a child who has never been dry)
  - Secondary (enuresis in a child who was previously dry)
  - Nocturnal (nighttime enuresis: bedwetting)
  - Diurnal (daytime: wetting clothes)
- More common in boys, nocturnal enuresis resolves spontaneously at 6 to 8 years of age in 15% of cases.

Risk Factors
- May have comorbidity with developmental disorders, learning problems, or behavioral difficulties

Prevention and Screening
- None

Assessment
- Urgency
- Acute discomfort
- Restlessness
- Urinary frequency

Management
- Conditioning therapy: Training the child to awaken with a stimulus initiated when the child voids (most effective)
- Retention control training: Child drinks lots of fluid and retains as long as possible to stretch the bladder
- Waking schedule: Parents wake the child during the night at intervals to void
- Medications: Tricyclic antidepressants, antidiuretics, and antispasmodics (least effective)

Outcomes and Follow-Up
- Education about the condition
- Encourage and support child and parents
- Teach parents side effects of medications

ATTENTION-DEFICIT DISORDER (ADD), ATTENTION-DEFICIT HYPERACTIVITY DISORDER (ADHD)

Description
Degrees of inattention, impulsivity, and hyperactivity beyond normal disturbances occurring at this stage of childhood development

Etiology
Multifactorial, including physiologic, genetic, and environmental factors

Incidence and Demographics
- 6% of school-age children; affects boys 3x as often as girls

Risk Factors
- Higher risk in children with family members with ADHD
- May be associated with substance abuse, learning disabilities, conduct disorders, depression, and antisocial personality disorders

Prevention and Screening
- None

Assessment
- Excessive impulsivity
- Inappropriately attentive
- Short attention span
- Hyperactivity may or may not be present
- Difficulty with organization

Management
- Therapy, counseling
- Medications: Ritalin, Cyclert, Dexedrine

Outcomes and Follow-Up
- Help plan activities to balance energy expenditure and quiet time
- Set realistic, attainable goals
- Structure situations for limited stimulation
- Consistent discipline
- Plan activities to ensure some success

EATING DISORDERS

Overweight and Obesity

Description
- The excessive accumulation of body fat relative to lean body mass is the most common nutritional concern of childhood.

Etiology
- Caloric intake that exceeds needs coupled with decreased activity

Incidence and Demographics
- In 2006, prevalence at 2 to 5 years was 12.4%; for 6 to 11 years, 17.0%, and for 12 to 19 years, 17.6% (Centers for Disease Control and Prevention, 2009)

Risk Factors
- 5% of obese children have an underlying medical condition (e.g., hypothyroidism, adrenal hypercorticoidism, hyperinsulinism, central nervous system damage)

Assessment
- Children with body mass index above the 95th percentile are obese and at high risk of remaining obese as adults; those at 85th to 94th percentile are overweight and at risk for remaining overweight as adults

Management
- Best management is prevention, as diet modification is difficult to maintain
- Increase physical activity
- Behavior modification
- Medications: appetite suppressants may be habit-forming and are not recommended
- Surgery: gastric bypass surgery is not recommended

Outcomes and Follow-Up
- Assess motivation
- Encourage personal responsibility
- Nutrition counseling (foods low in fat, smaller portions)

Anorexia Nervosa and Bulimia

Description
- *Anorexia:* Eating disorder characterized by refusal to maintain body weight within a normal range (American Psychiatric Association, 2000). Anorexic individuals feel hungry, but deny it.
- *Bulimia:* Eating disorder characterized by repeated binge-eating followed by purging through induced vomiting, laxatives, or excessive exercise.

Etiology
- Relentless pursuit of being thin
- Strongly dependent on parents
- Searching for sense of control
- Abnormalities of hypothalamic–pituitary and end-organ function

Incidence and Demographics
- Mainly occurs in White, middle–upper class females
- High achievers
- 0.5%–1% of young females

Risk Factors
- None

Prevention and Screening
- None

Assessment
- Self-imposed starvation
- Frequent strenuous exercise
- Social isolation
- Secondary amenorrhea
- Bradycardia
- Decreased blood pressure
- Hypothermia

Management
- Psychotherapy
- Family therapy
- Malnutrition reversal

Outcomes and Follow-Up
- Nutritional assessment
- Health interview
- Strengthen self-esteem
- Family support

SUBSTANCE ABUSE

(See also Chapter 7, Life Situations and Adaptive/Maladaptive Responses)

Description
Overindulgence in and dependence on a drug or other chemical, leading to effects that are detrimental to the individual's physical and mental health or the welfare of others.

Etiology
Most substance abuse begins with experimentation, is then used occasionally, and gradually becomes an integral part of a lifestyle.

Incidence and Demographics
- 4% of adolescents report daily use of alcohol
- 1%–2% of adolescents report regular use of "hard drugs" (Hockenberry & Wilson, 2009)

Risk Factors
- Parental substance abuse
- Child abuse/neglect
- Single-parent families
- Stressful life events
- Inadequate coping mechanisms

Prevention and Screening
- None

Assessment (varies depending on substance abused)
- Nausea, vomiting
- Slurred speech
- Poor coordination
- Hypertension
- Weight loss
- Flashbacks
- Hallucinations
- Gastritis
- Respiratory depression
- Coma
- Death
- Irreversible damage to central nervous system

Management
- Rehabilitation
- Foster healthy interdependent relationships

Outcomes and Follow-Up
- Foster feelings of self-worth
- Sensitivity to developmental transitions

DEPRESSION

Description
A psychiatric disorder that generally includes a state of unhappiness or hopelessness and manifests in many different ways in childhood, depending on developmental stage and language and cognitive development.

Etiology
- Acute: Usually temporary after an event such as death of a parent or close friend
- Chronic: Related to illness or disability

Incidence and Demographics
Approximately 3% to 5% (Shaffer et al., 1996)

Risk Factors
- Chronic illness such as diabetes
- Female gender
- Puberty
- Parental depression
- Neglect or abuse
- Socioeconomic deprivations
- Loss of loved one or loss of romantic relationship
- Anxiety disorder
- ADHD
- Smoking

Prevention and Screening
- None

Assessment
- Persistent feelings of hopelessness
- Dejection
- Poor concentration
- Lack of energy
- Inability to sleep
- Suicidal tendencies

Management
- Counseling
- Psychotherapy
- Family therapy
- Cognitive therapy
- Education about coping skills
- Environmental therapy
- Medications (tricycle antidepressants, selective serotonin reuptake inhibitors [SSRIs])

Outcomes and Follow-Up
- Careful history of child as depression may be difficult to assess
- Family education re: meds (take 2–4 weeks to reach therapeutic effect; monitor for side effects)

SUICIDE

Description
- Deliberate self-injury with intent to die
- Suicide ideation: Preoccupation with thoughts of committing suicide
- Suicide intent: Injury intended to result in death but unsuccessful

Incidence and Demographics
- Whites ages 15–24: 18.5% males, 3.3% females
- Blacks ages 15–24: 15% males, 2.2% females
- Hispanics ages 15–24: 13.4% males, 2.8% females (Murphy, 2000)

Risk Factors
- Depression
- Alcohol or drug use
- Impulsivity
- Feelings of guilt
- Body image problems
- Gender identity questions
- Difficult family situation
- Lack of effective social support

Prevention and Screening
- None

Assessment
- Ask adolescent screening questions (Greydanus & Pratt, 1995)
  - Do you consider yourself a happy person?
  - Have you ever been so upset you wanted to be dead?
  - Have you ever thought about hurting yourself?
  - Have you ever had a plan to hurt yourself?
  - Have you ever attempted to kill yourself?

Management
- Preventive care:
  - Counseling
  - Psychotherapy
  - Family therapy

Outcomes and Follow-Up
- Ensure safety
- Confidentiality may not be possible to honor for safety's sake
- Show of caring and understanding
- Express commitment
- Follow up with family, if needed

LOSS AND GRIEF/DEATH AND DYING

(See also Chapter 7, Life Situations and Adaptive/Maladaptive Responses)

Description
The concept "grief" is derived from a Latin word gravere, meaning to burden or to cause distress. Lindemann's (1944) seminal work noted that grieving persons display heightened irritability and anger, and may withdraw socially, despite efforts of others to support them. However, definitions continue to be vague and ambiguous. Bowlby's attachment theory (1969) refers to the state and quality of an individual's connections with others. A threat of loss typically results in anxiety and the actual loss usually leads to sorrow. Because grief has not been shown to progress in a rigid manner, it is described as a dynamic process with a broad range of feelings and reactions. Individuals may experience physical sensations, thoughts, behaviors, and feelings after a loss.

Etiology
To help a child dealing with death, nurses must be aware of the child's understanding and previous experience with death. The concept of death develops through stages according to a child's cognitive abilities. Death as irreversible, inevitable, and universal is not understood by many children until preadolescence, although the concept is certainly influenced by parental attitudes and explanations as well as personal experiences.

Incidence and Demographics
- While about 50,000 children in the United States die each year, children also are faced with grief associated with deaths of parents, friends, grandparents, or even pets

Risk Factors for Complicated Grief
- Inadequate support system or friendships
- Feelings of guilt
- Inability to talk about feelings
- History of depression or anxiety
- Violent or sudden death

Prevention and Screening
- None

Assessment
- Reactions may be physical, psychological, or cognitive
  - Frequent illness, overeating or undereating, insomnia
  - Antisocial behavior, depression, compulsions
  - Forgetfulness, difficulty concentrating
  - May be ongoing
- Influencing factors
  - Amount of social support
  - Prior positive coping skills
  - Open family communication style
  - Spiritual and religious beliefs
  - Anticipatory grief

Management
Going through grief is hard work and a process that takes time; in severe cases, cognitive–behavioral methods for symptoms and stress relief, along with interpersonal techniques to encourage reengagement with the world may be helpful

Outcomes and Follow-Up
- Be in touch with your own feelings
- Be compassionate and unafraid to show your caring and concern
- Provide anticipatory guidance of disease progression and dying process as parent(s) desire
- Seek opportunities to provide honest information, without being evasive and in a sensitive manner
- Encourage expression of feeling
- Provide support and active listening; use silence and presence
- Recognize that a child's serious illness affects the entire family system
- Encourage family's participation in child's care, including siblings and extended family members as desired
- Provide private area for parents and family members near child's bedside
- Assist parents in identifying and utilizing support systems

- Encourage family members directly involved in the patient's care to take care of themselves and to seek medical care when they fail to adequately care for themselves
- Facilitate parent's spiritual needs and rituals as desired
- Facilitate memory-making between child and family as desired (e.g., videotaping, scrapbooking)
- Identify and document patient, family, and caregiver needs related to anticipatory grieving (National Hospice and Palliative Care Organization, 2006).

CHILD ABUSE AND NEGLECT

(See also Chapter 7, Life Situations and Adaptive/Maladaptive Responses)

Description
One of the most significant social concerns affecting infants and children; may be classified as intentional physical abuse or neglect, emotional abuse or neglect, or sexual abuse

Etiology
A precise cause of abuse is unknown, but its etiology is influenced by parental characteristics, child characteristics, and environmental characteristics. It is the interaction among several factors that increases the risk for abuse.

Incidence and Demographics
- In the United States, approximately 800,000 to 1,000,000/year (U.S. Department of Health and Human Services, 2008)
  - Approximately 68% neglect
  - 20% physical abuse
  - 12% sexual abuse

Risk Factors
- Parents who were abused
- Socially isolated families
- Children of teen mothers
- Low self-esteem of parents
- Parents who use drugs
- Parents with poor understanding of typical childhood development
- Child's temperament
- Child's position in family
- Premature infants
- Children of a difficult pregnancy

Prevention and Screening
- None

Assessment

Physical
- Bruises on face, back, buttocks, torso
- Welts in regular patterns descriptive of objects used
- Burns on soles of feet, palms of hands
- Fractures such as spiral or dislocation, or in various stages of healing

Sexual
- Bruises, bleeding, lacerations of external genitalia
- Penile discharge
- Recurrent urinary tract infections

Management
- Prevention is best strategy
- Manage child's injuries or neglect

Outcomes and Follow-Up
- Protect child from further injury
- Mandatory reporting of even suspected child abuse
- Support child
- Support parents

HYPOTHERMIA

Description
Cooling of inner body core below 35° C or 95° F.

Etiology
Very young children with high BSA in relation to weight are at high risk

Incidence and Demographics
- Unusual with exception of trauma or accidental drowning

Risk Factors
- None

Prevention and Screening
- None

Assessment
- Variable respiratory rate
- Decreased intestinal motility
- Vigorous shivering or muscular rigidity
- Impaired speech and cognition
- Decreased metabolic rate
- Decreased oxygen uptake

Management
- Rewarming with warm humidified oxygen, IVs, dialysis
- Maintenance of ventilation
- Cardiac and renal monitoring
- Fluid and electrolyte replacement

Outcomes and Follow-Up
- Remove wet clothing
- Warm, high-caloric liquids if conscious
- Careful history of occurrence
- Monitor vital functions
- Education re: prevention of future occurrences

HYPERTHERMIA

Description
Body temperature exceeding set point, resulting from body creating more heat than it can eliminate

Etiology
Heat stroke, aspirin toxicity, hyperthyroidism

Incidence and Demographics
Though elevated temperatures are very common in children, they are most frequently associated with infections. True hyperthermia is primarily associated with heat stroke, aspirin toxicity when the body temperature exceeds the set point.

Risk Factors
- Aspirin poisoning
- Extremely hot environment

Prevention and Screening
- None

Assessment
- Metabolic rate increases 10% with each 1° C of hyperthermia and 3–5x with shivering.

Management
- Antipyretics do not help as they do with fever
    - Cooling measures with cooling blankets, cooling mattresses, or cool compresses
    - Tepid tub bath
    - Dry patient off and dress in lightweight pajamas
    - Stimulate circulation

REFERENCES

American Psychiatric Association. (2000). *Diagnostic and statistical manual of mental disorders* (4th ed.). Washington, DC: Author.

Barlow, S. E., & Dietz, W. H. (1998). Obesity evaluation and treatment: Expert committee recommendations. *Pediatrics, 102*(3), e29.

Birmaher, B., Rayan, N. D., Williamson, D. E., Brent, D. A., Kaufman, J., & Dahl, R. E. (1996). Childhood and adolescent depression: A review of the past 10 years. Part I. *Journal of the American Academy of Child & Adolescent Psychiatry, 35,* 1427–1439.

Bowlby, J. (1969/82). *Attachment and Loss. Volume 1: Attachment.* New York: Basic Books.

Centers for Disease Control and Prevention. (2000). Youth risk behavior surveillance: United States. *MMWR, 49*(SS05), 1–96.

Centers for Disease Control and Prevention. (2009). *Overweight and obesity: NHANES surveys (1976–1980 and 2003–2006).* Retrieved from http://www.cdc.gov/obesity/childhood/prevalence.html

Dietz, W. H., & Robinson, R. M. (1998). Use of the body mass index (BMI) as a measure of overweight in children and adolescents. *Journal of Pediatrics, 132*(2), 191–193.

Greydanus, D. E., & Pratt, H. D. (1995). Emotional and behavioral disorders of adolescence. *Adolescent Health Update, 8*(1), 1–8.

Hockenberry, M. J., & Wilson, D. (2009). *Wong's nursing care of infants and children* (8th ed.). St. Louis, MO: Mosby Elsevier.

Lindemann, E. (1944). Symptomatology and management of acute grief. *American Journal of Psychiatry, 101*(3), 141–149.

Lo, C. C., & Cheng, R. D. (2007). The impact of childhood maltreatment on young adults' substance abuse. *American Journal of Drug and Alcohol Abuse, 33*(1), 139–46.

Murphy, S. L. (2000). Deaths: Final data for 1998. *National Vital Statistics Report, 48*(11), 1–105,

National Child Traumatic Stress Network. (2004). *Fact sheet on children with developmental disabilities.* Retrieved from www.NCTSNet.org

National Hospice and Palliative Care Organization. (2006). *Standards of practice for hospice programs. Professional Development and Resource Series.* Alexandria, VA: Author.

Newacheck, P. W., & Halfon, N. (1998). Prevalence and impact of disabling chronic conditions in childhood. *American Journal of Public Health, 88*(4), 610–617.

Parkes, C. (1965). Bereavement and mental illness. *British Journal of Medical Psychology, 38,* 1–26.

Pilgrim, C. C., Schulenberg, J. E., O'Malley, P. M., Bachman, J. G., & Johnston, L. D. (2006). Mediators and moderators of parental involvement on substance use: A national study of adolescents. *Prevention Science, 7*(1), 75–89.

Shaffer, D., Gould, M. S., Fisher, P., Trautman, P., Moreau, D., & Kleinman, J. (1996). Psychiatric diagnosis in child and adolescent suicide. *Archives of General Psychiatry, 53,* 339–348.

U.S. Department of Health and Human Services. (2008). *Reports of incidence of child abuse.* Retrieved from www.hhs.gov

Westbrook, L. E., Silver, E. J., & Stein, R. E. (1998). Implications for estimates of disability in children: A comparison of definitional components. *Pediatrics, 101*(6), 1035–1030.

20

Health Maintenance, Promotion, and Wellness

Paula K. Yim Chiplis, PhD, RN, CPNP, and Mary Jo Gilmer, PhD, MBA, CNS, CNL

Health maintenance, promotion, and wellness include physical, cognitive, emotional, and social dimensions.

- *Health maintenance* refers to activities that prevent disease or injury, thus preserving health.
- *Health promotion* refers to activities that promote well-being or health according to an individual's potential. Thus, individuals with disabilities can be healthy if they adapt to their condition.
- *Wellness* refers to a healthy balance of body, mind, and spirit, resulting in an overall feeling of wholeness or well-being.
- *Health supervision* refers to services that focus on growth and development, screening, health promotion at key developmental stages, and services that prevent diseases and injuries and treat diseases. Health supervision is the core of primary care pediatrics and general pediatrics.

Table 20–1. Age, Weight, Height, and Developmental Issues

Age Group	Age	Weight	Head Circumference	Physical Development Issues
Newborn	Birth–1 week	2,700–4,000 g (6–9 lbs)	33–35 cm (13–14 in)	Transition to extra-uterine well-being
Infant	1 week–1 yr		35–48 cm (14–19 in)	Developmental milestones
Toddler/ Preschooler	2–4 yrs	• 14.5 kg (32 lbs) @ 3 yrs • 16.5 kg (36.5 lbs) @ 4 yrs • 18.5 kg (41 lbs) @ 5 yrs	48–52 cm (19–20.5 in)	Gross motor, fine motor skills
School Age	5–12 yrs			Cognitive development
Adolescent	13–18 yrs			Sexual development, menarche

IMMUNIZATIONS

A rapid decline in the number of infectious diseases during the 20th century has been a dramatic benefit of the widespread use of immunizations. The recommended schedule begins during infancy. Visit http://www.cdc.gov/vaccines/recs/schedules/child-schedule.htm for the Center for Disease Control and Prevention's recommendations for immunization schedules.

Preterm infants should receive full doses of vaccines at the appropriate chronologic age.

Hepatitis B
Preservative-free Hep B (Recombivax HB, no mercury) is now available.
* *Reaction:* Few side effects
* *Nursing Responsibilities:* Administer IM in vastus lateralis of newborns or in deltoid for older infants and children. First dose should be given within 12 hours of birth. Can be administered simultaneously at separate site with DTaP, MMR, and Hib. Should not be given to children allergic to baker's yeast.

Hepatitis A
* *Reaction:* Few side effects
* *Nursing Responsibilities:* No severe reactions. Erythema at site. Second dose should be given at least 6 months after first dose.

Diphtheria
* *Reaction:* Fever within 24–48 hours; soreness, redness, and swelling at site. Behavioral changes (e.g., fussy, fretful, anorexia, unusual crying).
* *Nursing Responsibilities:* Withhold for encephalopathy ≤ 7 days after previous DTaP. Advise of potential side effects and have parents call for neurological symptoms and temperature ≥ 40.5° C (104.9° F). Boosters given every 10 years.

Tetanus

- *Reaction:* Same as for diphtheria, plus urticaria and malaise. May have delayed onset and/or lump at site that lasts weeks or months but eventually disappears.
- *Nursing Responsibilities:* Boosters every 10 years after DTaP/DTP vaccine series

Pertussis

- *Reaction:* Acellular pertussis vaccine has fewer local and systemic side effects (such as redness at site, fever, and irritability) than the whole-cell pertussis vaccine.
- *Nursing Responsibilities:* Same as for tetanus, plus loss of consciousness, convulsions, inconsolable crying episodes, generalized or focal neurologic signs, systemic allergic reaction

Polio

- *Reaction:* Inactivated poliovirus vaccine (IPV) is now recommended because of the rare risk of vaccine-associated paralysis. This change increased cost and the number of injections necessary.
- *Nursing Responsibilities:* Four doses are needed and only IPV is used in the United States. Contraindicated if anaphylactive response to neomycin or streptomycin.

Measles

Vitamin A decreases the morbidity and mortality of measles.
- *Reaction:* To the live, attenuated vaccine, anorexia, malaise, rash, and fever 7–10 days after
- *Nursing Responsibilities:* Advise parents of side effects and use of acetaminophen for fever

Mumps

- *Reaction:* To the live, attenuated vaccine, brief, mild fever
- *Nursing Responsibilities:* Should not be administered to infants < 12 months old because maternal antibodies can interfere with immune response. Recommended for all individuals born after 1957 who are at risk for the disease.

Rubella

Mild disease in children but causes congenital disease, cataracts, sensorineural deafness, and congenital heart defects in the newborn if contracted in the first trimester. When contracted intra-uterine, may also cause mental retardation, cerebral palsy, sudden hearing loss, glaucoma, progressive encephalitis, and increased incidence of type 1 diabetes.
- *Reaction:* To the live, attenuated vaccine, fever, lymphadenopathy, mild rash lasting 1–2 days, arthritis, arthralgia, and paresthesia of hands and fingers 2 weeks after vaccination
- *Nursing Responsibilities:* Advise of side effects, especially of time delay of joint pain, assuring them that symptoms will disappear. May cross placental barrier and the immunization should not be given to pregnant women. Contraindicated with known immunodeficiency. Recommend acetaminophen if needed for fever or discomfort.

Haemophilus influenzae Type B (Hib)

- *Reaction:* Mild pain and redness, low-grade fever
- *Nursing Responsibilities:* Advise parents of side effects and use of acetaminophen for fever

Varicella (Chickenpox, VZV)
- *Reaction:* To live attenuated vaccine, local soreness or swelling, fever, rash
- *Nursing Responsibilities:* Advise of side effects. Recommend acetaminophen if needed. Should not be given to infants prior to 12 months of age. Has been shown to be effective for at least 11 years. Contraindicated with HIV, known immunodeficiency, pregnancy.

Pneumonococcal
- *Reaction:* Local tenderness, fever, anorexia
- *Nursing Responsibilities:* Not recommended for children 2, 4, 6 and 12–15 months of age

Influenza
Recommended annually for children ≥ 6 months of age with risk factors (asthma, cardiac disease, HIV, diabetes, and sickle cell disease)
- *Reaction:* Soreness, fever, aches
- *Nursing Responsibilities:* Administer in early fall before flu season begins and repeat annually. Do not administer to children with hypersensitivity to eggs. FluMist may be given nasally in two doses 4 weeks apart in individuals 2–49 years old instead of vaccine.

Meningococcal
- *Reaction:* MCV4: Pain at site, fever, headache, fatigue, chills, anorexia, vomiting, diarrhea, rash. MPSV4: Pain at site, redness, fever, urticaria, wheezing, rash.
- *Nursing Responsibilities:* Explain benefits, especially in adolescents and young children. Contraindicated in person allergic to diphtheria toxoid or latex.

Human Papilloma Virus (HPV)
- *Reaction:* Local irritation, fever
- *Nursing Responsibilities:* Recommended for female children and adolescents to prevent HPV-related cervical cancer. Three doses needed. Contraindicated with pregnancy or hypersensitivity to yeast.

Inactivated vaccines may result in limited side effects such as local tenderness, erythema, fever, drowsiness, and irritability. These responses usually occur within a few hours or days. Live vaccines such as MMR may result in unfavorable reactions 30 to 60 days after administration.

Administration
Immunizations may be given IM or Sub-Q (MMR, Varicella, and meningococcal). The needle length should be selected dependent on the amount of a child's sub-Q tissue. Needle gauge should be as small as possible to deliver the medication; 25–30-gauge needles are least painful, but larger diameter may be necessary for viscous medications. Ensuring the correct dose of a medication given is a shared responsibility of the practitioner and the nurse. Children may unexpectedly react with severity to some drugs and care should be taken to monitor children carefully.

ANTICIPATORY GUIDANCE/PATIENT SAFETY
(Home, Hospital, and Community)

The meaning of health needs to be modified to adapt to changing populations.

Falls

While falls are more common after an infant has learned to roll over (~4 mos), they can occur at any age. Caregivers should be encouraged to get in the habit of raising side rails all the way and to never leave a child on a changing table unattended, even when restrained. Infant seats, high chairs, swings, and walkers also present challenges to prevent falls. Never leave an unattended infant on a raised surface: the safest place may be the floor. To prevent falls once an infant is mobile, gates should be used at the tops and bottoms of any stairs. Furniture should be kept away from windows.

Poisoning

Because of their curiosity and impulsivity, young children are particularly vulnerable to poisoning. The most frequent cause is improper storage in the home. Toddlers are very quick and can swallow a whole bottle of aspirin in seconds. Parents should be advised to call a Poison Control Center before initiating an intervention. Generally, first aid for various types of poisoning:

- *Caustics/Corrosives (Drano, lye):* Do not induce vomiting, because a substance that burns on the way down can burn on the way back up. The child needs emergent care with a lavage tube to suction out the poison.
- *Hydrocarbons (gasoline, cleaning solutions):* Treat like caustics or corrosives and do not induce vomiting. These substances are usually excreted through the lungs and may cause respiratory depression.
- *Medications:* Syrup of ipecac is no longer recommended because it may result in prolonged vomiting. In its place, activated charcoal is an odorless, tasteless, fine black powder that adsorbs many compounds and may be mixed with soda for a child to drink.
- *Metals:* As there is no normal excretory mechanism to rid the body of metal ingestion, chelation therapy is typically used to bind with the metal for rapid and safe excretion.

Injury Prevention
Vehicular Safety

Motor vehicle accidents remain the leading cause of accidental death in children <9 years of age (CDC, 2007). Car seats for infants and young children are mandatory in all states. The safest location for an infant is in the rear seat, facing backwards.

Toy Safety

Though toys are integral to a child's play, they can be hazardous and it is the nurse's responsibility to ensure toy safety in a hospital setting. If a child is receiving oxygen therapy, electrical or friction toys are contraindicated as sparks may cause the oxygen to ignite. Toys with small parts should be avoided in children < 3 years of age. Latex balloons are also not appropriate because a young child may choke on a piece of latex if the balloon breaks.

Adolescent Issues

Sexuality

Anticipatory guidance can help prevent unfortunate choices teens may make that negatively affect their futures. Many children report never having been informed about puberty development and sexuality issues (Omar, McElderry, & Azkharia, 2003). Education should consist of normal anatomy and physiology, using correct terminology adolescents can understand. They also need to know about biological processes and mechanics of conception so they can make informed decisions about intimate relationships and their future.

Smoking and Drug Use

The prevalence of smoking has decreased in recent years, but continues to be the most common cause of preventable death. While the dangers of smoking prevail at any age, it is particularly important to prevent smoking at a young age because of its addictive nature. Although experimentation with illegal drugs is widespread (American Academy of Pediatrics [AAP], 2005), most teens do not become high-risk users. Nurses can play an important role in administering educational programs to prevent smoking and drug use as part of holistic anticipatory guidance toward a healthy lifestyle.

COMMUNITY-BASED SCREENING AND RESOURCES

Newborn Universal Screening for Metabolic Disorders and Hemoglobinopathy

At birth or 1 week. Screening for conditions varies by state and results must be documented.

Hearing

At birth or in the first month; a normal result must be documented by the 2-month visit or further evaluation is needed. Congenital hearing loss should be identified before 3 months of age. Hearing should be evaluated at the 4-year, 5-year, 8-year, and 10-year visits.

Vision

Screening should be done at an early age and at regular intervals (AAP, 2003). Infants and children should be assessed for visual acuity, peripheral vision, color vision, and ocular alignment.

- *Visual acuity:* In infants, a check for light perception and a test of ability to follow an object are used. Fixed pupils, strabismus, nystagmus, or setting sun sign all indicate visual loss or other serious concerns. A common test for visual acuity in children is the Snellen chart, with lines of letters of decreasing size. If a child is unable to read letters, a tumbling E test can be used and a child is asked to point the direction the E is facing. Typically by the time an infant is 3 to 4 months, she or he has the ability to view one visual field with both eyes simultaneously.
- *Peripheral vision:* Useful with older children is checking the ability to fix eyesight on a space directly in front, and then moving an object such as a pencil and asking the child to indicate when she or he can no longer see it.

- *Color vision:* Tests for color vision use a series of pictures composed of spots of one color in the background and an object in the foreground composed of spots of a color often confused with the background. Almost 10% of White males are assessed as having poor color vision.
- *Ocular alignment:* Typically, by the time infants are 3 to 4 months old they can see a visual field with both eyes simultaneously. However, with strabismus (cross-eye), one eye deviates. The weak eye may become lazy over time. The corneal light reflex test is used to determine alignment if a light falls symmetrically within each pupil when the light shines directly into the child's eyes. Another test is the cover test where a child is asked to look at an object and then one eye is covered and movements of the uncovered eye are observed.

Anemia
At 4 months, hemoglobin and hematocrit for preterm, low birth weight, and those fed non–iron-fortified formula. At 12-month, 2-year, 3-year, and all other visits, risk assessment questions asking about limited access or avoidance of high-iron foods, e.g., vegan diet

Oral Health
At 6 months, question feeding practices (e.g., bottle in bed) and examine teeth. At 12 months, refer to dentist with visits every 6 months.

Lead
At 12 months and 2 years, test those in high-prevalence areas or with Medicaid insurance. Ask environmental risk questions at 6 months, 9 months, 12 months, 18 months, 2 years, 3 years, 4 years, 5 years, and 6 years: Does the child live in a building built before 1950, or built before 1978 and recently renovated? Test refugee children 6 months to 16 years old upon entering the United States and repeat for those 6 months to 6 years of age 3 to 6 months after permanent placement.

Tuberculosis
A tuberculin skin test (TST) is a screening test used to determine if a child has been infected in the tubercle bacillus. Universal screening is no longer recommended by AAP; screening is done only when a child is at high risk for contracting the disease.

Autism
Screen at 18-month and 2-year visits with an autism-specific screening tool.

Blood Pressure
Annually beginning at 3-year visit. Prior to 3 years old, monitor according to risk conditions such as prematurity, very low birth weight, renal disease, congenital heart disease, or other neonatal complications.

Body Mass Index (BMI) and Weight for Length
Assess weight, length, and weight for length every visit from birth until the 18-month visit. Beginning at 2-year visit, BMI for age percentile according to standing height.

Dyslipidemia

- *Fasting lipoprotein profile* (total cholesterol, LDL, HDL, and triglycerides): Once in late adolescence.
- *Dyslipidemia risk assessment:* At 2-year, 4-year, 6-year, 8-year, and 10-year visits and then annually according to risk for coronary artery disease due to family history, BMI, or health behaviors.
- *Fasting lipid profile:* For all persons with a BMI ≥ 85th percentile, even if no other risk factors are present (Barlow, 2007).

Sexually Transmitted Infections (STI)

- For sexually active youth, annual screen for chlamydia and gonorrhea.
- Selective HIV screen for sexually active youth with positive response to risk assessment (injection drug users, men who have sex with men, women with unprotected sex with multiple partners, persons who exchange sex for money or drugs, persons treated for sexually transmitted infection, bisexual, partners of those with HIV).

Pregnancy

Sexually active females who report late menses or amenorrhea.

Cervical Dysplasia

Females 3 years after onset of sexual activity or at age 21.

Alcohol or Drug Use

Risk assessment at every adolescent visit (Have you ever had an alcoholic drink? Have you ever used marijuana or another drug to get high?). A positive response should trigger the use of a screening tool, such as CRAFFT, designed for use with teens in primary care settings.

Developmental/Behavioral Assessment

At every visit

Scoliosis

At 5th and 7th grade

Denver Developmental Screening Tool

Denver Developmental Screening Tool (DDST II) is a revised developmental screening tool with 125 items used to determine relative areas of advancement or delay in development.

BARRIERS TO CARE

Access

May be a concern related to socioeconomic conditions, physical constraints, mental status, transportation, finances, lack of insurance, or many other barriers to care.

Availability

Individuals living in rural areas may have limited availability of services, but limited access to the services that do exist may be related to social standing, economic status, and poor health (Powers & Faden, 2006).

Culture

Barriers to care may be related to lack of family support, the need for the patient to be primary caregiver for others whose needs they put first, transportation difficulties, or mistrust of Western medicine.

Health Literacy

Defined in Healthy People 2010 as: "The degree to which individuals have the capacity to obtain, process, and understand basic health information and services needed to make appropriate health decisions."

REFERENCES

American Academy of Pediatrics. (2006). Tobacco, alcohol, and other drugs: The role of the pediatrician in prevention, maintenance, and identification of substance abuse. *Pediatrics, 115*(3), 812–815.

American Academy of Pediatrics Committee on Practice and Ambulatory Medicine and Bright Futures. (2007). Steering Committee recommendations for preventive pediatric health care. *Pediatrics, 120*(6), 1376.

Ball, J. W., & Binder, R. C. (2008). *Pediatric nursing: Caring for children* (4th ed.). Upper Saddle River, NJ: Pearson Prentice Hall.

Barlow, S. E. (2007). Expert committee recommendations regarding the prevention, assessment, and treatment of child and adolescent overweight and obesity: Summary report. *Pediatrics, 120*(Suppl 4), S164–S192.

Centers for Disease Control and Prevention. (2006). Prevention of hepatitis A through active or passive immunization. *MMWR, 55*(RR-7), 1–23.

Centers for Disease Control and Prevention. (2007). Fatal injuries among children by race and ethnicity—United States, 1999–2002. *MMWR, 56*(SS-5), 1–16.

Hockenberry, M. J., & Wilson, D. 2007. *Wong's nursing care of infants and children* (8th ed.). St. Louis, MO: Mosby Elsevier.

Omar, H., McElderry, D., & Zakharia, R. (2003). Educating adolescents about puberty: What are we missing? *International Journal of Adolescent Medicine and Heath, 15*(1), 79–83.

Powers, M., & Faden, R. (2006). *Social justice.* New York: Oxford University Press.

Rank, M. R. (2005). *One nation underprivileged: Why American poverty affects us all.* New York: Oxford University Press.

Spenceley, S. M., Reutter, L., & Allen, M. N. (2006). The road less traveled: Nursing advocacy at the policy level. *Policy, Politics and Nursing Practice, 7*(3), 180–194.

INTERNET RESOURCES

www.aap.org: American Academy of Pediatrics (AAP).
   Organization of physicians committed to physical, mental, and social health for all infants, children, adolescents, and young adults.

www.cdc.gov/vaccines: Advisory Committee on Immunization Practices (ACIP within CDC).
   Provides education for public and healthcare providers, school requirements, vaccine laws.

www.medicaid.gov: Medicaid.
   A state-administered program available to low-income individuals and families who fit into an eligibility group. Payments are sent directly to healthcare providers.

21

Management and Leadership

Karen Corlett, MSN, RN-BC, CPNP-AC/PC, PNP-BC

Pediatric nurses may be in management roles or be managed by other nurses. Each pediatric nurse has an opportunity to be a leader: at the individual unit or hospital, or at the community or national level, advocating for pediatric patients, pediatric health care and policy, and pediatric nursing.

PRINCIPLES OF MANAGEMENT

Leadership Styles
Autocratic
- Power lies with leader
- Leader makes decision and informs group
  - Group without options

Democratic
- Group comes to decision
- Leader facilitates group member involvement and decision-making

Laissez-faire
- Leader does not direct group
- Group may not be functional without leader
- Work may not be accomplished

Reactionary
- Leader is not change-directed
- Leader deals with situations after problems occur

Transformational
- Leader empowers members to create change by creating a shared vision
- Driving forces are organizational goals

Principles of Effective Leadership
- Model expected behavior
- Inspire a vision for improvement
- Challenge the process at all levels
  - Encourage thinking outside the box
  - Don't accept current thinking or processes as the only way
- Enable others
  - Current change processes may confine those with great ideas
- Encourage those you manage
  - Get to know professional goals and personal drives

Change Theories
Transtheoretical Model
PRECONTEMPLATION
- Denial and blaming common
- Feel change is not needed

CONTEMPLATION
- Need for change recognized
- Fear, anxiety, and ambivalence about actual change

PREPARATION
- Planning for change
- Exploration of options
  - Process of change
  - What change is actually necessary, needed, or wanted

ACTION
- Actual change occurs, may impact several areas
  - Behavior and attitudes
  - Structure and personnel
  - Process and work flow
  - Endpoint and measures of success

MAINTENANCE
  • Change is continued
  • Change is not a linear process
  • Individuals cycle up and down through the stages of change

TERMINAL STAGE
  • Previous behavior no longer desirable
  • Persons see new behavior/process/endpoint as the normal

Organizational Change
BARRIERS TO CHANGE
  • Personnel
    – Opposite of own interest
    – Assumptions/inaccuracies about effect of change
    – Do not value the proposed change
    – Change seen as unnecessary
    – Work stress does not leave energy for change
  • Systems
    – Stable systems are resistant to change

FORCES PROMOTING CHANGE
  • Personnel
    – Agree with need for change
    – Generation of, or agreement with, idea for the change
    – Change reduces workload
    – Idols and peers agree with change
  • Systems
    – Change decreases work
    – Pilot of change with open evaluation of process/outcomes
    – Change implemented with enthusiasm by leadership team

Conflict Resolution
Goals
• Resolution of dispute while meeting the needs of all parties
• Satisfaction through compromise rather than concession

Methods of Conflict Resolution
• Active listening
  – Reflecting, restating, summarizing
• Mediation
  – Third-party involvement in negotiation, with goal of compromise that is agreeable to both parties
• Arbitration
  – Third-party involvement as decision-maker; both parties may be legally bound by decision of arbitrator
• Litigation

Supervision and Delegation
- Nurses may be in the situation of supervising or delegating tasks to licensed or unlicensed personnel
- Stay within the state's nurse practice act
  - Nurse responsible for knowing which nursing tasks may be delegated
- Supervision and training of new nurses and new employees
  - Education on policies and procedures
  - Task-oriented as new nurses
  - Progression from direct supervision to resource for questions
  - Promotion of critical thinking skills
  - Case-based scenarios to promote critical thinking
  - Case studies and simulations

ORGANIZATIONAL STRUCTURE

Mission Statement
- Written documentation of the purpose of the organization
  - Range from one sentence to multipage documents
- Should be the driving force of the organization
  - Goals
  - Commitments
  - Values

Institutional Policy
Employee Management
- Illness and vacation
- Hiring and firing
- Counseling and disciplinary action

Patient Care
- Frequency of vital signs during administration of blood products
- Care of a central line
- Obtaining blood cultures

Standards of Care
- Family-centered care model
- Asthma care model
- Pathway for care of a child with community-acquired pneumonia

Chain of Command
- Accessible document that delineates the chain of command within an organization
- Appropriate pathway of escalation for problems or concerns
  - Escalation stops when satisfactory answer obtained
  - Sample issues
    - Nurse feels patient assignment is inappropriate or unsafe
    - Nurse feels harassed by another employee
    - Nurse feels disciplined unjustly

- Example for a bedside nurse
  - Self → charge nurse → shift supervisor or head nurse → nursing department director → nursing division director → chief nursing officer
  - If still unsatisfied, nurse may escalate outside of workplace to state nurses organization

PROFESSIONAL DEVELOPMENT

Employer Requirements
- Yearly requirements
  - Health and safety
    - Fire safety
    - Tuberculosis skin testing
    - Equipment operations and functioning
    - Security of patient information
    - Disaster awareness
- Ability to practice
  - Evaluations
    - Peers
    - Supervisors
    - Assessment for presence of complaints

Self-Development
- Up-to-date licensure
- Continuing education programs
  - Conferences
  - Self-study programs
  - Development and presentation of programs
- Certifications
  - Basic life support
  - Specialty certifications
- Professional organizations
  - Membership
  - Involvement
    - Committee work
    - Task forces
    - Office holder

REFERENCES

Kouzes, J. M., & Posner, B. Z. (2003). *A leadership challenge.* San Francisco: Pfeiffer.

Potts, N. L., & Mandleco, B. L. (Eds.). (2007). *Pediatric nursing: Caring for children and their families* (2nd ed.). Clifton Park, NY: Tomson.

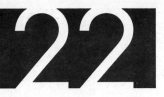

Research

Paula K. Yim Chiplis, PhD, RN, CPNP

STEPS OF THE RESEARCH PROCESS

- Identify a problem that can be studied
- Review the literature
- Define the theoretical framework
- Ask the research question or formulate the hypothesis
- Design the study
  - Identify the population, sample, variables, and methods of measurement
  - Build in appropriate controls to minimize bias
- Get institutional review board (IRB) approval
- Conduct the study
- Collect data
- Design database and enter data
- Analyze and interpret data
- Disseminate findings

USE OF RESEARCH IN PRACTICE

- There is a delay of 17 years before new knowledge is used in practice (Clancy, 2003)
- Only 60% of American patients with chronic diseases receive recommended care (Schuster et al., 1998)

EVIDENCE-BASED PRACTICE

Evidence-based practice (EBP) is more than applied science. It is nursing practice that is based on research findings, the consensus of experts, available resources, and patient preference to optimize patient outcomes. It de-emphasizes opinion, unsystematic clinical experience, intuition, and traditional practice. The randomized controlled trial (RCT) design is the most valid type of evidence.

Why EBP now?
- Growth of information
- Delay in implementing new knowledge
- Decline in knowledge of best care
- Sophisticated consumer pressure

Steps of EBP
- Identify an EBP question
- Search for evidence
- Critically evaluate the evidence
- Develop recommendations for practice
- Integrate the evidence into practice
- Measure outcomes to evaluate effectiveness or improved patient outcomes

CLINICAL PRACTICE GUIDELINES

Clinical practice guidelines define standards of care and help decision-making about specific diseases. They are based on clinical evidence and expert consensus.
- A *clinical pathway* is a method for managing a defined group of patients in a period of time. A clinical pathway explicitly states the goals and key elements of care based on evidence-based medicine (EBM) guidelines, best practice, and patient expectations.
- *Knowledge translation* is the use of research findings in clinical practice. It is a nonlinear process that involves not only research findings but also new knowledge that is created from the dynamic interaction of the people/groups who come together to solve health problems. Knowledge of translation methods include clinical pathways, audit and feedback, academic detailing, reminders, and local opinion leaders. These initiatives are instituted at the level of a particular hospital or agency with respect to a certain condition.

- *Best practice in nursing* is today's popular phrase that refers to the use of interventions and techniques that are based on research and known to promote higher quality of care. It is a generic phrase that isn't equivalent to EBN, which is a more rigorous concept. With the explosion of valuable practice-related reports, methods used by many nurses in the past, such as attending conferences, networking with colleagues, and reading professional journals, can barely keep pace with potentially important research.

REFERENCES

Clancy, T. R. (2003). The art of decision-making. *Journal of Nursing Administration, 33*(6), 343–349.

Hockenberry, M. J., & Wilson, D. (2007). *Wong's nursing care of infants and children* (8th ed.). St. Louis: Mosby Elsevier.

Schuster, M. A., McGlynn, E., & Brook, R. H. (1998). How good is the quality of health care in the United States? *Milbank Quarterly, 76,* 517–563.

Stetler, C. B., Brunell, M., Giulano, K. K., Morsi, D., Prince, L., & Newell-Stokes, V. (1998). Evidence based nursing and the role of nursing leadership. *Journal of Nursing Administration, 28*(7/8), 45–53.

University of Iowa, The John A. Hartford Center of Geriatric Nursing Excellence. (2008). *Best practices.* Retrieved from http://www.nursing.uiowa.edu/hartford/nurse/best_practice.htm

23

Legal and Ethical Issues

Karen Corlett, MSN, RN-BC, CPNP-AC/PC, PNP-BC

Legal definitions vary by state law. This chapter is intended not to delineate laws, but as a reference for concepts related to legal questions and ethical dilemmas.

GUIDELINES FOR THE PRACTICE AND DELIVERY OF HEALTH CARE

Federal Requirements
- Medicaid and Medicare requirements
  - Definitions of appropriate care, treatment, billing
- Health Insurance Portability and Accountability Act (HIPAA)
  - Privacy of patient information
- Emergency access to care without regard to race, gender, or ability to pay

Regulatory Requirements
- Federal, state, or local guidelines or statutes, such as:
  - The Joint Commission (formerly JCAHO)
    - Implements and evaluates practices for the improvement of patient safety
    - Provides accreditation to hospitals that meet criteria
      - Marker of safe practices
      - Accreditation necessary for Medicare reimbursement

– Clinical Laboratory Improvement Amendments (CLIA)
  • Describe safe and appropriate laboratory policies
  • Provide certification for compliant clinical laboratories
– Centers for Disease Control and Prevention
  • Requirements and regulations for reporting and tracking of contagious diseases
  • State health departments may have stricter or looser reporting criteria

Professional Nursing Practice
• Term "registered nurse" protected as to definition and use
• Licensure:
  – State-by-state regulation of the registered nurse
  – Grants permission to practice the profession of nursing within the state
  – Regulatory board charged with ensuring a minimum level of safety to the public
  – Many states part of a "compact" to improve portability of nurses from state to state without undergoing relicensing procedures
    • Each state in the compact accepts the nursing licensure of other states within the compact
• Certification:
  – National recognition of expertise within a particular specialty by a certifying body
    • Requirements for acquisition of certification
    • Requirements for maintenance of professional certification
  – Recognition of excellence, but not authority to practice

Nurse Practice Acts
  • State definition of the legal aspects of the practice of nursing within that state
  • It is the nurse's responsibility to read, understand, and stay within his or her state nurse practice act
  • Violation of nurse practice acts can result in disciplinary action

Standards of Practice
  • ANA-SPN-NAPNAP *Pediatric Nursing: Scope and Standards of Practice* (2008)
    – Sixteen standards describing the process and responsibilities for both generalist and advanced practice nurses who care for pediatric patients and their families The standards and scope include:
      · Clinical components of the nursing process
      · Evaluation of nursing process and professional practice
      · Quality
      · Education and research
      · Leadership
      · Teamwork and communication
      · Advocacy
  • Standards of Professional Performance for the Pediatric Nurse
    – Systematically evaluates the quality and effectiveness of pediatric nursing practice
    – Evaluates her or his own nursing practice in relation to professional practice standards and relevant statutes and regulations
    – Acquires and maintains current knowledge in pediatric nursing practice

- Contributes to the professional development of peers, colleagues, and others
- Makes decisions and takes actions on behalf of children and their families that are determined in an ethical manner
- Collaborates with the child, family, and healthcare providers in providing client care
- Uses research findings in practice
- Considers factors related to safety, effectiveness, and cost in planning and delivering care

- Other international, national, specialty organization, institutional, or practice-related guidelines for practice such as:
  - American Nurses Association Code of Ethics for Nurses with Interpretative Statements
  - CDC Guidelines for Immunization Practices
  - Society of Pediatric Nurses statement on Safe Staffing Practices
  - Institutional policies such as frequency of vital signs during administration of blood products
    - Unit policies such as placement of patients on cardio-respiratory monitoring devices

REIMBURSEMENT

- Most registered nurses do not bill directly for their services
- Anyone involved in billing is responsible for awareness of the billing process and mandatory reporting of unlawful practices
  - How the charge is generated
  - How the bill is prepared
  - Who is billed for the care
  - Where the money is distributed once received
  - HIPPA protection throughout the billing process
- Medicaid and Medicare as the gold standard for billing requirements
  - Documentation of care
    - Adequate for fee charged
  - Appropriate level of care billed for
    - Underbilling and overbilling both illegal
    - Can not "unbundle" care
      - For example, cardiac surgeon must charge to repair Tetralogy of Fallot rather than billing for VSD closure and repair of pulmonary stenosis
    - Cannot "double dip"
      - If employed by department of nursing, cost of nursing care is typically rolled into the daily room charge; a nurse cannot also submit a separate bill for a dressing change
      - Those employed by another entity may be able to bill for procedures, care, or consultation

AUTHORITY FOR DECISION-MAKING

- Adults have authority for their own medical decision-making
  - Definition of adult varies by state and by situation
    - Reaching age definition of legal adult (18 years)
    - A minor who is legally married, has joined the military, lives on his or her own and is financially self-supporting, or has given birth may be considered an adult by legal definitions
  - Incapacitated adults (illness, injury, or incompetence)
    - Next of kin or delineated medical decision-maker to give authorization for health care
- Those not of legal age or situation must have consent of a parent or guardian to receive health care
  - Physical custody of child does not imply legal custody
    - Many complex situations
      · Divorce
      · Remarriage
      · In-process adoptions
      · Incapacitated or injured parents/guardians
      · Children in protective custody
    - Consult legal counsel for assistance if any question
  - Special situations where minor children may have ability to receive care without parental consent (state-by-state definitions)
    - Pregnancy care or prevention
    - Testing and treatment for sexually transmitted diseases
    - Treatment for drug or alcohol use/abuse
    - Suspected or substantiated abuse or neglect of a minor child
    - Emergent situation in which two physicians agree delay of care would adversely affect child

Informed Consent
- Responsibility of healthcare provider to inform parent/guardian/patient of the proposed treatment, risks, benefits, and alternatives in terms they can understand
  - Opportunity for questions and clarifications
  - Parent/guardian can refuse to give consent to some or all of proposed treatments
  - Nurses typically sign as witness to event
    - Role as advocate for patient/family understanding
    - Consult state law for definition of responsibility

Assent of Minor Children
- Minor agrees to allow procedure
- Age-appropriate explanation of procedure
- May be requirement for assent in pediatric research studies

Limitation of Life-Saving Treatment
- Involve judicial system if medical team believes treatment is beneficial to child and parent/guardian denies
  - Support for family and child if court intervenes to order treatment

- Limitation of care
  - Mechanism for advance directive for those classified as legal adults
  - Facilitate discussion with patient/parent for those with chronic illness and known risk of death
    - Age and developmentally appropriate approach to discussion
    - Involve child life for ongoing support and therapies
  - Limitation of resuscitation discussed with parent/guardian

ETHICAL DILEMMAS

- Patient care situation with no clear-cut correct answer
- Typically is difference of opinion on appropriate care
  - Difference can be between:
    - Providers
    - Parents
    - Parents and providers
    - Hospital/agency and providers or parents
    - Insurance coverage and any of the above

Principles of Ethical Decision-Making

Respect for Autonomy
- The ability of persons to make their own decisions in a manner appropriate for themselves
- Respect of each individual's own decision

Beneficence
- Helping others is primary motivator

Nonmaleficence
- Avoidance of harm is driving force

Justice
- Allocation of resources
- Respect of rights
- Respect of morals
- Respect of beliefs

Ethical Theories

Deontology
- Rules and principles guide decision-making
- Concepts of right and wrong
- Consequences not the major decision-driver

Teleology
- Outcome as most important event
- Outcome justifies the means

Virtue
- Intent is the most important concept
- Outcome is trumped by the intent of the decision-maker

Care
- The wishes or assumed wishes of the patient are of utmost concern

Utilitarianism
- The good of society is of utmost concern
- The benefit of the outcome is compared to the relative cost of the action
  - Cost can be defined as monetary, pain, suffering, risk to others, energy expenditure, etc.

NURSING RESPONSIBILITIES

- Explore own ethical viewpoint
- Professional relationship with patient and family
  - ANA statement
- Support of patient and family during ethical discussions
- Escalating ethical dilemmas through appropriate channels
  - Hospital ethics committees
  - Legal counsel

REFERENCES

American Nurses Association. (2001). *Code of ethics for nurses with interpretive statements.* Washington, DC: Author.

Betz, C. L. (2008). Pediatric nursing: Scope and standards of practice: A unified professional effort. *Journal of Pediatric Nursing, 23*(2), 79–80.

Brannigan, M. C., & Boss, J. A. (2001). *Healthcare ethics in a diverse society.* Mountain View, CA: Mayfield Publishing.

Gillon, R. (1994). Medical ethics: Four principles plus attention to scope. *British Medical Journal, 309*(6948), 184–188.

Husted, G. L., & Husted, J. H. (2001). *Ethical decision making in nursing and healthcare: The symphonological approach* (3rd ed.). New York: Springer.

International Council of Nurses. (2001). *The ICN code of ethics for nurses.* Geneva, Switzerland: Author.

Potts, N. L., & Mandleco, B. L. (Eds.). (2007). *Pediatric nursing: Caring for children and their families* (2nd ed.). Clifton Park, NY: Tomson.

Society of Pediatric Nurses. (2007). *The Society of Pediatric Nurses position statement: Safe staffing for pediatric patients.* Retrieved from https://www.pedsnurses.org/component/option,com_docman/ Itemid,0/task,doc_view/gid,69

Review Questions

1. While working in a well-child clinic, a nurse is asked by a new mother how to best encourage development of social skills in her young infant. Which of the following responses is the nurse's best reply, based on Erikson's theory of psychosocial development?
   a. Enroll the infant in a play group
   b. Allow the infant to learn self-amusement
   c. Meet the baby's physical needs, cuddle, and comfort the infant
   d. Show the mother the rooting reflex

2. A nurse is in charge of a pediatric unit in an acute care facility. Considering typical growth and development, which of the following considerations is most important in making a room assignment for a 10-month-old infant?
   a. May have underlying fear of body mutilation
   b. Will want to be with infants of the same age
   c. Regression is a normal response
   d. Consistent caregiver presence

3. A 12-month-old baby is being evaluated for growth and development. The baby weighed 6 pounds at birth and now weighs 9 kg. What is the correct analysis of the data?
   a. Baby is gaining less weight than expected
   b. Baby is probably being overfed
   c. Baby should be evaluated for failure to thrive
   d. Baby is gaining weight at an expected rate

4. Play is a child's work. Which of the following statements best describes a 2½-year-old's play preferences?
   a. Likes to play games that have rules
   b. Shares toys and plays cooperatively with other toddlers most of the time
   c. Imitates observed adult behaviors
   d. Paints and draws independently

5. As a nurse, you are expected to provide anticipatory guidance to new parents. One of the mothers in your clinic states that her 2-year-old child doesn't seem to want to eat much at mealtime anymore. The mother is quite concerned. How can the nurse best respond?
   a. Your child's brain is developing and he must be made to eat meat each day.
   b. Try offering small amounts of food frequently instead of providing three meals a day.
   c. If your child doesn't want to eat, give milk in a bottle to be sure he gets enough calories.
   d. It is normal for the appetite to decrease, but be sure he has plenty of carbohydrates for brain development.

6. You are a bedside nurse on an acute care unit at a children's hospital. A 2-year-old child, Benjamin, is off the unit having a chest X-ray when the parents approach the nurse and say, "We're going home for the night now." What is the nurse's best response?
   a. Have a good night; we'll see you in the morning.
   b. I'll tell Benjamin you had to leave.
   c. Go ahead and leave. I'm sure Benjamin will be asleep when he comes back from radiology.
   d. Please wait to tell Benjamin good-bye before you leave.

7. The nurse is observing the activities of young children. Which of the following indicates appropriate general development in a 5-year-old?
   a. Learning to draw the figure of a person
   b. Obeying two-step commands
   c. Identifying colors and shapes
   d. Riding a tricycle in the playroom

8. Considering Piaget's theory of cognitive development, which task should the nurse expect of a typically developing 10-year-old?
   a. Makes up complicated games with imaginary friends
   b. Engages in parallel play
   c. Asks simple hypothetical questions and explores possible solutions
   d. Learns beginning reading skills

9. An adolescent has been recently diagnosed with diabetes mellitus. She is having difficulty adhering to diet and medication therapy. Which of the following is the most important factor influencing compliance in adolescents?
   a. Abstract reasoning ability
   b. Family support and attention
   c. Reactions of peer group
   d. Nurse's empathy with the adolescent

10. In sequencing a physical examination on a 16-month-old, which assessment should be performed at the end of the exam?
    a. Genitalia
    b. Heart and respiratory rates
    c. Lower extremities
    d. Tympanic temperature

11. Which pain assessment scale would be the best choice for a 9-month-old?
    a. CRIES
    b. FACES
    c. FLACC
    d. Numeric 1–10

12. Which assessment finding is unexpected and qualifies as a cause of concern?
    a. Abdominal, rather than diaphragmatic, breathing in a 36-month-old
    b. Bow-leg stance in a standing 18-month-old
    c. Closed anterior fontanel in a 6-month-old
    d. Small, painless, movable cervical lymph node in a 12-month-old

13. The mother of a 3-month-old breastfed infant tells the nurse that her son is too small because he is at the 10th percentile on a standardized growth chart. The nurse's best response is:
    a. Don't worry, in a few months he'll get up to the 50th percentile.
    b. His birth weight was also at the 10th percentile, so he should be at the 30th now.
    c. It is time to start supplementing with formula after each feeding.
    d. Your son's place on the chart is within normal limits.

14. A mother reports her infant has been vomiting for 24 hours, unable to hold anything down. The infant has just been admitted to an emergency room at a children's hospital. Even before the lab work is available, the nurse should observe for signs of:
    a. hyperactivity
    b. acidosis
    c. alkalosis
    d. tetany

15. When a child is having a severe asthma attack, the most common acid–base imbalance is:
    a. Respiratory acidosis related to impaired respirations and increased carbonic acid
    b. Metabolic alkalosis related to excessive production of acid metabolites
    c. Metabolic acidosis related to the kidney's inability to compensate for increased carbonic acid
    d. Respiratory alkalosis related to accelerated respirations and loss of carbon dioxide

16. A 3-year-old child has been admitted to the hospital for surgery to correct congenital megacolon. Preoperatively, enemas are ordered to cleanse the bowel. Keeping in mind fluid and electrolyte balance, the nurse should use:
    a. Hypertonic phosphate
    b. Isotonic saline
    c. Tap water
    d. Soap suds

17. Young children are more prone than adults to develop otitis media because their Eustachian tubes are:
    a. Longer
    b. More rigid
    c. More slanted
    d. Wider

18. Which statement best describes hearing loss in a child? Conductive hearing loss:
    a. improves with a cochlear implant.
    b. is an inherited type of hearing loss.
    c. may accompany otitis media with effusion.
    d. results from auditory nerve damage.

19. A nurse should question which of the following medications ordered for a child with hyphema, accumulation of blood in the anterior chamber?
    a. Acetaminophen (Tylenol)
    b. Aminocaproic acid (ACA, Amicar)
    c. Ibuprofen (Motrin)
    d. Timolol maleate (Timoptic-XE)

20. The infant with acute gastroenteritis may be encouraged to drink:
    a. Apple juice
    b. Breast milk
    c. Jell-o™ water
    d. Chicken broth

21. The definitive diagnostic test for Hirschsprung disease is:
    a. Anorectal manometry
    b. MRI scan
    c. Radiography
    d. Rectal biopsy

22. Before surgery, nursing care for the newborn with tracheoesophageal fistula and esophageal atresia includes
    a. Continuous or intermittent suction to clear secretions
    b. Measurement of abdominal girth every hour
    c. Supine position under radiant warmer
    d. Small, frequent feedings of glucose water

23. A 2-year-old with intussusception is scheduled for surgery in 1 hour. The crying, hungry child passes a soft brown stool. The nurse should
    a. administer an antispasmodic medication
    b. call the surgeon to report the stool passage
    c. place a warm compress on the child's abdomen
    d. send the specimen to the lab for analysis

24. A toddler with iron deficiency anemia is given an oral iron supplement. What advice should the nurse give the parent?
    a. A mild antacid will lessen the accompanying stomach discomfort
    b. Brush the child's teeth after giving the medication
    c. Do not give citrus juice within 1 hour of iron administration
    d. Expect the child's stools to appear slightly rust-colored

25. Which of the following is an accurate statement about hydroxyurea therapy for sickle cell anemia?
    The medication is:
    a. administered to increase hemoglobin F level
    b. most effective if started in infancy
    c. started after first vaso-occlusive crisis
    d. used primarily for sequestration crisis

26. Which of the following is indicative of the most common manifestation of hemophilia?
    a. Black, tarry stools
    b. Hematuria
    c. Knee stiffness
    d. Severe headache

27. Which is true about the treatment of acute myeloid leukemia (AML) in children?
    a. Cranial radiation is necessary
    b. Maintenance therapy lasts at least 2 years
    c. Stem cell transplant is done after the first remission
    d. There is no effective treatment for this type of leukemia

28. Which guideline for childbearing women who are HIV-positive is true?
    a. Antiretroviral therapy is stopped during pregnancy to protect the fetus
    b. Breastfeeding is avoided because it is a route of transmission
    c. Newborns do not need to be tested until signs of infection appear
    d. Vaginal delivery is preferred because there is less bleeding

29. HIV-positive children are at risk of developing *Pneumocystis carinii*. Which medication is given as prophylaxis for this organism?
    a. Azithromycin (Zithromax)
    b. Hyperimmune globulin (VZIG)
    c. Isoniazid (INH)
    d. Trimethoprim/sulfamethoxazole (Bactrim)

30. Teaching for the adolescent with systemic lupus erythematosus (SLE) should stress the importance of:
    a. limiting intake of foods high in calcium.
    b. minimizing sun exposure at all times.
    c. rigidly restricting exercise activities.
    d. using sodium supplements during the summer.

31. A diagnosis of bacterial meningitis is supported by which cerebrospinal fluid finding?
    a. Decreased glucose level
    b. Extremely low white blood cell count
    c. Low level of protein
    d. Presence of red blood cells

32. A child with cerebral palsy is started on baclofen therapy. Which statement made by the nurse most accurately describes baclofen administration?
    a. "Baclofen is never administered orally."
    b. "It directly enters the spinal column."
    c. "I will show you how to do the daily injection."
    d. "The most likely side effect is spastic movement."

33. To decrease the risk of neural tube defects, it is recommended that a multivitamin containing folic acid
    be given to
    a. all women of childbearing age.
    b. expectant mothers over age 40.
    c. women of all ages.
    d. women testing positive for pregnancy.

34. The most likely diagnosis for a 10-year-old girl who only vomits in the morning when she gets out of bed is
    a. brain tumor
    b. encephalitis
    c. lyme disease
    d. viral meningitis

35. A Pavlik harness is ordered for initial treatment of an infant with developmental dysplasia of the hip (DDH). To prevent skin irritation, the nurse advises the child's parents to
    a. apply a mild lotion, keeping the skin lubricated.
    b. remove the harness for 10 minutes every 3–4 hours.
    c. tuck an undershirt under the harness for padding.
    d. use a small amount of powder to absorb perspiration.

36. Legg-Calvé-Perthes disease (LCPD) involves lack of circulation and necrosis of the
    a. head of the femur
    b. malleolus of the ankle
    c. patella of the knee
    d. talus of the foot

37. The nurse reminds parents of a child being treated with serial casting (Ponseti method) for congenital clubfoot to return to have the first cast replaced in:
    a. 1 week
    b. 1 month
    c. 2 months
    d. 6 months

38. When caring for a child in a long leg cast, the nurse notes that the child has a pedal pulse and is able to move the toes, but has slight blue discoloration and coolness of the toes. Which nursing action is most appropriate?
    a. Assure parent that this is normal and administer pain medication
    b. Cover the toes with a towel and recheck in 15 minutes
    c. Elevate leg above the level of the heart using pillows
    d. Notify the physician immediately

39. The nurse encourages a child to wear sunglasses in the house. This child probably has:
    a. Fifth disease (erythema infectiosum)
    b. Rubella (German measles)
    c. Rubeola (measles)
    d. Varicella (chickenpox)

40. Skin care for a 2-year-old with eczema includes:
    a. Fabric softener to keep clothing comfortable
    b. Heavy lubrication with cream such as Eucerin
    c. Topical hydrocortisone each evening to prevent scratching
    d. Warm, moist compresses for 20 minutes before bed

41. A 5-year-old girl comes to the emergency room of a small, rural hospital after being burned. The nurse should prepare the family for the child's transfer to a larger city with a pediatric burn center if the burn
    a. appears intensely red and radiates heat.
    b. consists of red, painful skin covering the girl's back.
    c. covers the anterior thigh and has blisters and swollen tissue.
    d. involves the palm of one hand and has white, brown, charred areas.

42. Management of acne in the adolescent girl includes
    a. avoiding all facial cosmetics.
    b. concealing forehead acne with clean hair.
    c. daily gentle cleansing with mild soap.
    d. regular use of antibacterial skin cleanser.

43. Upon referral from his second-grade teacher, a 7-year-old has been diagnosed with attention-deficit disorder with hyperactivity and cylert 37.5 mg/day has been ordered. The nurse discussing the child's treatment with the child's mother should emphasize that it is important to:
    a. point out to her son that he can control his behavior if he tries.
    b. avoid imposing too many rules because the added frustration could make the disorder worse.
    c. monitor the effect of the medication of her son's behavior.
    d. tutor her son in the subjects that are troublesome.

44. For a child diagnosed with autism, the hope of leading a normal, productive life is:
    a. dependent on early diagnosis.
    b. looked upon with caution related to the clinical manifestations of autism, which affect many areas of functioning.
    c. often related to the child's overall temperament.
    d. part of anticipatory guidance regardless of the child's level of functioning.

45. Choose the best reason for the ability to play "peek a boo" is
    a. Development of 20/20 vision
    b. Object permanence
    c. Depth perception
    d. Head control

46. When teaching parents of a 6-month-old infant how to prevent falls, the nurse should emphasize that at this age, an infant can generally:
    a. Crawl long distances
    b. Sit up
    c. Roll over
    d. Walk short distances while holding onto furniture

47. It is contraindicated to give live virus vaccines such as measles to children who are receiving steroids, antineoplastics, or radiation therapy because these children may
    a. be unlikely to need the protection of an immunization during their short life span.
    b. have had the disease or have been immunized previously.
    c. have an allergy to rabbit serum, which is an additive to live vaccines.
    d. be susceptible to getting the disease because of a depressed immune response.

48. A 5-year-old child is preparing to start kindergarten. The child has received all of the primary immunizations, and the father asks which immunizations the child still needs. Which of the following is the nurse's best response?
    a. DTaP, IPV, and MMR
    b. Measles and rubella
    c. IPV and Hep B
    d. DTaP and tuberculin test

B

Answers to the Review Questions

1. **Correct Answer: C.** An infant's stage of psychosocial development is trust versus mistrust. Meeting the baby's physical and emotional needs will help the development of trust.

2. **Correct Answer: D.** Separation anxiety typically becomes prominent around 6–8 months, and a 10-month-old baby will be more comfortable with a consistent caregiver.

3. **Correct Answer: D.** Infants typically double birth weight by 6 months and triple it by 12 months.

4. **Correct Answer: C.** Toddlers engage in parallel play and like to imitate others.

5. **Correct Answer: B.** Toddlers eat small amounts of food and are picky, fussy eaters.

6. **Correct Answer: D.** A toddler typically trusts parent more than hospital staff and though the 2-year-old may cry when the parents leave, it is best to be honest and it will be an easier adjustment for the child if parents are the ones to inform the child that they are leaving for the night.

7. **Correct Answer: A.** A 3-year-old can obey a 2-step command, identify colors and shapes, and ride a tricycle, but it is not until 4–5 years that a child learns to draw the figure of a person.

8. **Correct Answer: C.** Concrete operations are forming at 7–11 years. The 10-year-old child progresses from making judgments based on observation to judgments based on reason.

9. **Correct Answer: C.** Identity formation in adolescence is based on the adolescent's interactions with others, particularly friends and peers.

10. **Correct Answer: D.** Tympanic temperature is the most invasive. Heart and respiratory rates should be done early in the exam with the child quiet and on the parent's lap. Toddlers, unlike older children, are not concerned about private areas. Checking lower extremities is often fun for a mobile toddler.

11. **Correct Answer: C.** FLACC may be used for children 2 months through 7 years. CRIES is indicated for children 0–6 months, FACES for those over 3 years, and numeric for those older than 9 years.

12. **Correct Answer: C.** The anterior fontanel should close at 12–18 months. Children use abdominal breathing until about 6 years of age. Bow-leg appearance is normal for children younger than 3 years. Small, painless, movable nodes are common findings in children.

13. **Correct Answer: D.** The child who falls between the 5th and 90th percentiles is within normal limits. Children usually closely follow the same percentile throughout their lifetimes, so would not be expected to jump from the 10th to the 30th to the 50th.

14. **Correct Answer: C.** With excessive vomiting, hydrogen ions are lost through the emesis (hydrochloric acid), which results in metabolic alkalosis related to an excess of base bicarbonate.

15. **Correct Answer: A.** In an asthma attack, a child has restricted ventilation, which limits the ability to blow off carbon dioxide. Water then combines with the carbon dioxide to form carbonic acid (H_2CO_3), resulting in respiratory acidosis.

16. **Correct Answer: B.** Isotonic saline is neither hypertonic or hypotonic, and minimizes the risk of a change in osmotic pressure with resulting imbalance of intracellular and extracellular fluid and electrolytes.

17. **Correct Answer: D.** A young child's Eustachian tube is wider, shorter, and straighter, with less developed cartilage.

18. **Correct Answer: C.** Conductive hearing loss may accompany otitis media with effusion, when fluid in the middle ear blocks the transmission of sound. Sensorineural hearing loss may improve with cochlear implant, is inherited in 50% of cases, and may be due to damage of the auditory nerve.

19. **Correct Answer: C.** Ibuprofen (Motrin), a nonsteroidal anti-inflammatory, might increase the bleeding. Acetaminophen may be used for pain without a bleeding risk. Aminocaproic acid is ordered to prevent secondary bleeding and timolol maleate to decrease intraocular pressure.

20. **Correct Answer: B.** Breast milk is the most nutritionally balanced and well-tolerated choice. Apple juice and Jell-o water have high carbohydrate content and low electrolyte content, which won't replace lost electrolytes. Meat broth has an excessive amount of sodium and inadequate carbohydrate content.

21. **Correct Answer: D.** A rectal biopsy would show absence of ganglion cells, essential for confirmation of the diagnosis of Hirschsprung disease. Anorectal manometry would show the absence of internal anal sphincter relaxation that occurs, but is not diagnostic. MRI and radiography would show dilated bowel, which again is not diagnostic.

22. **Correct Answer: A.** The correct answer is continuous or intermittent suction to clear secretions that accumulate in the esophageal pouch. The esophagus is not connected to the stomach, so air does not accumulate to expand the abdomen. The infant should be placed in an upright or prone position with the head elevated at least 30° to prevent aspiration. NPO status is maintained or fluid will enter the trachea.

23. **Correct Answer: B.** The nurse should call the surgeon to report the stool passage, because this indicates resolution of the intussusception and surgery is no longer necessary. The child is likely irritable due to NPO preoperative status, which will change when surgery is cancelled. There is no need for medication, warm compress, or lab analysis at this time.

24. **Correct Answer: B.** The parent should brush the child's teeth after giving the medication because iron supplements can stain teeth. Antacids decrease the absorption of iron. Citrus juice enhances absorption. The stools may turn dark green or black, not rust-colored.

25. **Correct Answer: A.** Hemoglobin F level is the normal hemoglobin that does not sickle like hemoglobin S. The medication is given to adolescents and adults who have more than three episodes of vaso-occlusive crisis per year. It is not used for sequestration when large quantities of blood pool in the spleen.

26. **Correct Answer: C.** Knee stiffness is a sign of hemarthrosis, bleeding into a joint, which is the most common manifestation of hemophilia. Black, tarry stools indicate bleeding in the gastrointestinal tract. Hematuria means bleeding in the renal system. Headache is a sign of intracranial hemorrhage. All of these are less common than hemarthrosis.

27. **Correct Answer: C.** Stem cell transplant done after the first remission is the treatment of choice. Cranial radiation and maintenance therapy are used in acute lymphoblastic leukemia (ALL), but not in AML. Chemotherapy and stem cell transplant can be effective in AML.

28. **Correct Answer: B.** Breastfeeding should be avoided because it is a route of transmission. Antiretroviral therapy is continued during pregnancy. Newborns should be tested as soon as possible so treatment can begin if the result is positive. Cesarean section is preferred over vaginal delivery to minimize the infant's contact with maternal fluid.

29. **Correct Answer: D.** Trimethoprim/sulfamethoxazole (Bactrim) should be used as prophylaxis for Pneumocystis carinii. Isoniazid is given for Mycobacterium tuberculosis to children with a positive TB skin test or TB contact. Hyperimmune globulin is given to prevent varicella (chickenpox) after exposure.

30. **Correct Answer: B.** The rash of SLE is especially sensitive to ultraviolet light, including sunlight and uncovered fluorescent light. Supplemental calcium and vitamin D is often necessary to prevent osteoporosis, a common side effect of the corticosteroids used to treat SLE. Regular exercise is beneficial in preventing the osteoporosis and coronary artery disease that often occurs with SLE. Another complication of SLE is renal involvement with hypertension, which is treated by a low-sodium diet.

31. **Correct Answer: A.** Decreased glucose level supports a diagnosis of bacterial meningitis. In bacterial meningitis, the WBC count and protein level are elevated. The red cells occur during lumbar puncture and are not considered diagnostic.

32. **Correct Answer: B.** Baclofen may be given intrathecally with an implanted pump. There is an oral form. There is no need for daily injection. It is given to decrease spasticity.

33. **Correct Answer: A.** All women of childbearing age should receive a multivitamin containing folic acid. Neural tube defects occur early in pregnancy, before a woman of any age may even realize that she is pregnant or have a pregnancy test. Multivitamins are not recommended for all females.

34. **Correct Answer: A.** Change in position from lying to upright characterizes the vomiting that occurs with a brain tumor. The vomiting that might occur with the others is more frequent and sporadic.

35. **Correct Answer: C.** Lotion would make the area too moist and powder would be drying, both increasing the risk for irritation. The harness is worn continuously for the first 6 weeks and then part-time for another 6 weeks.

36. **Correct Answer: A.** LCPD involves only the femur, not the other structures.

37. **Correct Answer: A.** Casts are replaced each week for 4–8 weeks.

38. **Correct Answer: B.** Although coolness and discoloration may indicate impaired circulation, the presence of pedal pulse and movement make this unlikely. The toes may be cool due to environmental temperature. Reassuring the parent, administering pain medication, and elevating the leg will not warm the toes. There is no need to notify the physician at this time.

39. **Correct Answer: C.** Rubeola (measles) is characterized by photophobia, which usually does not accompany the other communicable diseases.

40. **Correct Answer: B.** Daily emollient relieves the dry, scaly skin of eczema. Fabric softener often irritates eczema. Topical corticosteroids are only used for short periods of time. The overheating that could happen with warm compresses would also irritate the skin.

41. **Correct Answer: D.** Major burns involve more than 20% of total body surface area or are full thickness burns of any extent. The palm is less than 20%, but the appearance indicates a full thickness burn. The first response does not give enough information to assess either extent or depth of the burn. Red, painful skin of the back is superficial and less than 20%. Blisters and swollen tissue of anterior thigh is partial thickness and less than 20%.

42. **Correct Answer: C.** Oil-free facial cosmetics that are labeled "noncomedogenic" are safe. Hair gets progressively oilier throughout the day and should be kept off the forehead. Antibacterial cleansers are not necessary and may cause excess drying of the skin.

43. **Correct Answer: C.** In monitoring her son's behavior, the mother assists the physician in determining the effectiveness of the medication.

44. **Correct Answer: B.** Evidence indicates that hope for normal productive functioning in individuals diagnosed with autism should be guarded, especially if there are delays in language development.

45. **Correct Answer: B.** Around 10 months of age, an infant develops a sense of object permanence and understands that an object may still be there and will search for it, even when it is out of view.

46. **Correct Answer: C.** Infants typically learn to roll over by 4–5 months and are at risk of falling if elevated and unattended.

47. **Correct Answer: D.** Use of steroids results in depression of the immune response. Antineoplastic drugs destroy lymphatic tissue and bone marrow, where antibody production and other immune responses occur. Radiation also may alter immune responses

48. **Correct Answer: A.** For a child 4–6 years old, immunizations required by law include DTaP; IPV; and measles, mumps, and rubella.

Index

About the Authors

Paula K. Yim Chiplis, PhD, RN, CPNP, is a coronary critical care nurse at Holy Cross Hospital in Silver Spring, Maryland. She was a rehabilitation pediatric nurse practitioner and taught pediatric clinicals at Johns Hopkins.

Karen Corlett, MSN, RN-BC, CPNP-AC/PC, PNP-BC, has been a nurse involved in the care of pediatric patients for more than 20 years. She has always worked in pediatric tertiary care facilities providing direct patient care. Karen started working on the inpatient ward, caring for infants with a wide range of medical and surgical problems; she then specialized in pediatric cardiac surgery, working with the cardiac surgery team caring for patients throughout their cardiac surgical experience. She finished her nurse practitioner degree and transitioned to a role in the pediatric ICU as a nurse practitioner. She now works as a PNP in a cardiac ICU in Dallas, Texas.

Karen lectures in local baccalaureate nursing programs in the Dallas area and is a frequent lecturer in acute care PNP programs around the country. She holds national certification as a primary care and acute care PNP. She has authored a chapter on the cardiovascular system in a text for pediatric nurse practitioners. She lectures at local, regional, and international programs on a variety of topics related to cardiology and cardiac surgery.

Mary Jo Gilmer, PhD, MBA, APN, CNL, is a graduate of Michigan State University's School of Nursing. She began her career in nursing at Children's Memorial Hospital in Chicago, Illinois while she completed her MSN at the University of Illinois. She worked as a clinical specialist in pediatric cardiovascular surgery before receiving a Commonwealth Fund Executive Nurse Fellowship to pursue an MBA at Queens University. Dr. Gilmer earned her PhD in nursing at the University of North Carolina–Chapel Hill.

Before coming to Vanderbilt, Dr. Gilmer was on the faculty at Queens University. Throughout her career, she has received numerous awards for her research and teaching expertise. She has been a leader in several international healthcare projects, including initiatives in Belize, Uganda, China, Italy, and Ecuador.

Beginning in 2002, Dr. Gilmer's research and practice have focused on enhancing care of children with life-threatening conditions. Her work at Monroe Carell Jr. Children's Hospital at Vanderbilt involved establishment of an interdisciplinary team to develop research initiatives, clinical services in palliative care, education and training, and support services in palliative care. Her current research is focused on parent and sibling bereavement after a child dies from cancer and parent–child communication about cancer.

Clara J. Richardson, MSN, RN-BC, received a BSN from DePaul University, Chicago, and an MSN degree from Indiana University. She is a clinical associate professor at Purdue University School of Nursing. She also serves as the director of the Center for Nursing History, Ethics, and Human Rights located in the School of Nursing and as the site coordinator for the School of Nursing Community Level Training Team of the Brazelton Touchpoints Center.

Professor Richardson has taught pediatric nursing, both lecture and clinical, to undergraduate students for 29 years. She also teaches an undergraduate course on children's health care for the Child Development and Family Studies Department.

Professor Richardson has been certified as a pediatric nurse by the American Nurses Credentialing Center since 1997. She is a member of the Delta Omicron Chapter of Sigma Theta Tau International, the Society of Pediatric Nurses, Nurses Christian Fellowship, and the American Association for the History of Nursing.